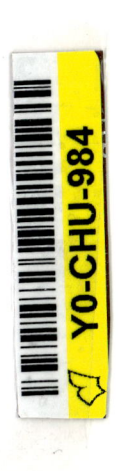

Manual of Clinical Child Psychiatry

Manual of Clinical Child Psychiatry

Edited by

Kenneth S. Robson, M.D.

*Professor of Psychiatry,
Tufts University School of Medicine; and
Associate Division Chief for Training (Child Psychiatry),
New England Medical Center Hospitals*

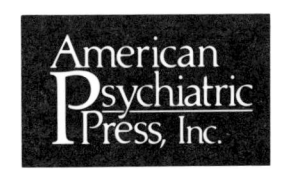

American Psychiatric Press, Inc.

1400 K Street, N.W.
Washington, DC 20005

Note: The authors have worked to ensure that all information in this book concerning drug dosages, schedules, and routes of administration is accurate as of the time of publication and consistent with standards set by the U.S. Food and Drug Administration and the general medical community. As medical research and practice advance, however, therapeutic standards may change. For this reason and because human and mechanical errors sometimes occur, we recommend that readers follow the advice of a physician who is directly involved in their care or the care of a member of their family.

Books published by the American Psychiatric Press, Inc., represent the views and opinions of the individual authors and do not necessarily reflect the policies and opinions of the Press or the American Psychiatric Association.

Cover design by Sam Haltom
Text design by Richard E. Farkas
Typeset by Harper Graphics
Printed by Semline, Inc.

Copyright © 1986 Kenneth S. Robson
ALL RIGHTS RESERVED
Manufactured in the United States of America

First printing - May 1986
Second printing - February 1987
Third printing - January 1988
Fourth printing - November 1988

Library of Congress Cataloging in Publication Data

Main entry under title:

Manual of clinical child psychiatry.

  Includes bibliographies and index.
  1. Child psychiatry. I. Robson, Kenneth S. [DNLM: 1. Child Psychiatry. 2. Mental Disorders—in infancy & childhood. WS 350 M294]
RJ499.M2635   1986   618.92'89   85-26869
ISBN 0-88048-037-8 (pbk.)

Contents

Contributors vii
Preface xi

PART 1   DIAGNOSTIC ASSESSMENT

Chapter 1	Introduction to Diagnostic Assessment *Kenneth S. Robson, M.D.*	3
Chapter 2	Diagnostic Assessment: Technical Considerations *Kenneth S. Robson, M.D.*	21
Chapter 3	Physical and Neurological Examinations and Laboratory Studies *P. S. B. Sarma, M.B., B.S.* *William D. Singer, M.D.*	35
Chapter 4	Psychological Testing *Sid Mondell, Ph.D.* *Terrell Clark, Ph.D.*	65
Chapter 5	Formulation, Differential Diagnosis, and Treatment Planning *Kenneth S. Robson, M.D.*	103

PART 2   APPROACHES TO TREATMENT

Chapter 6	Introduction to Treatment *Kenneth S. Robson, M.D.*	113
Chapter 7	Therapeutics I: The Psychotherapies *Kenneth S. Robson, M.D.*	119

Chapter 8	Therapeutics II: Intensive Milieu Therapy, Behavior Therapy, and Hypnosis *Virginia S. Villani, M.D.* *Janet Gillmore, Ph.D.* *Joae G. Brooks, M.D.*	131
Chapter 9	Therapeutics III: Pharmacotherapy *Barbara J. Coffey, M.D.*	149
Chapter 10	Emergencies I *Judith Robinson, M.D.*	185
Chapter 11	Emergencies II: Sexual Abuse and Rape in Childhood *Maria Sauzier, M.D.* *Catherine Mitkus, LIC.S.W., M.S.W.*	213

PART 3 CONSULTATION AND RELATED CLINICAL PROBLEMS

Chapter 12	Consultations *Ourania Madias, M.D.* *Kenneth S. Robson, M.D.*	243
Chapter 13	Forensic Child Psychiatry *Joseph J. Jankowski, M.D.* *William P. Monahan, J.D.* *Stephen Porter, M.D.*	251
Chapter 14	Adoption and Foster Care *Steven L. Nickman, M.D.* *Marie Armentano, M.D.*	269
Chapter 15	Infant and Toddler Psychiatry *Margaret P. Gean, M.D.*	289
Chapter 16	Genetic Issues in Child Psychiatry *Bonnie D. Cummins, M.Ed.* *Kenneth S. Robson, M.D.*	303

Index	313

Contributors

Marie Armentano, M.D.
Instructor in Psychiatry,
Harvard Medical School; and
Staff, Child and Adolescent Psychiatry Unit,
Massachusetts General Hospital,
Boston, Massachusetts

Joae G. Brooks, M.D.
Assistant Clinical Professor of Psychiatry,
Harvard Medical School; and
Private Practice of Child Psychiatry,
Brookline, Massachusetts

Terrell Clark, Ph.D.
Staff Psychologist,
Children's Hospital Medical Center,
Boston, Massachusetts; and
Lecturer, Department of Child Study,
Tufts University,
Medford, Massachusetts

Barbara J. Coffey, M.D.
Assistant Clinical Professor of Psychiatry,
Tufts University School of Medicine; and
Director, General Psychiatry (Child) and
   Psychopharmacology (Child) Clinic,
New England Medical Center Hospitals,
Boston, Massachusetts

Bonnie D. Cummins, M.Ed.
Boston, Massachusetts

Margaret P. Gean, M.D.
Assistant Professor of Psychiatry,
Tufts University School of Medicine; and
Director, Infant/Toddler Clinic,
New England Medical Center Hospitals,
Boston, Massachusetts

Janet Gillmore, Ph.D.
Staff Psychologist,
Harvard Community Health Plan,
Wellesley, Massachusetts

Joseph J. Jankowski, M.D.
Associate Clinical Professor of Psychiatry,
Tufts University School of Medicine; and
Associate Division Chief for Ambulatory and Community Services (Child Psychiatry),
New England Medical Hospitals,
Boston, Massachusetts

Ourania Madias, M.D.
Faculty Member,
Harvard Medical School; and
Staff Psychiatrist, In-Patient Child Psychiatry Service,
Children's Hospital Medical Center,
Boston, Massachusetts

Catherine Mitkus, LIC.S.W., M.S.W.
Clinical Instructor in Child Psychiatry,
New England Medical Center Hospitals; and
Director of the Governor's Special Commission on Violence Against Children,
Executive Office of Human Services,
Commonwealth of Massachusetts,
Boston, Massachusetts

William P. Monahan, J.D.
Associate Clinical Professor of Psychiatry,
Tufts University School of Medicine; and
Director, Behavior Problems Clinic,
New England Medical Center Hospitals,
Boston, Massachusetts

Sid Mondell, Ph.D.
Instructor in Psychiatry,
Tufts University School of Medicine; and
Director of Psychology Training,
New England Medical Center Hospitals,
Boston, Massachusetts

Steven L. Nickman, M.D.
Clinical Instructor in Psychiatry,
Harvard Medical School; and
Medical Director for Children's Services,
New Bedford Area for Human Services, Inc.,
New Bedford, Massachusetts

Stephen Porter, M.D.
Instructor in Psychiatry,
Tufts University School of Medicine; and
Consultant, South Boston Court Clinic,
Boston, Massachusetts

Judith Robinson, M.D.
Assistant Professor of Psychiatry and Director,
In-Patient Child Psychiatry Service,
New England Medical Center Hospitals,
Boston, Massachusetts

Kenneth S. Robson, M.D.
Professor of Psychiatry,
Tufts University School of Medicine; and
Associate Division Chief for Training (Child Psychiatry),
New England Medical Center Hospitals,
Boston, Massachusetts

P. S. B. Sarma, M.B., B.S.
Associate Professor and Director of Child Psychiatry,
Department of Psychiatry and Behavioral Sciences,
University of Health Sciences/The Chicago Medical School,
Chicago, Illinois

Maria Sauzier, M.D.
Clinical Instructor in Psychiatry,
Harvard Medical School; and
Consultant to Department of Pediatrics and Sexual Abuse Team,
Cambridge Hospital,
Cambridge, Massachusetts

William D. Singer, M.D.
Faculty Member,
Harvard Medical School; and
Associate Chief of Pediatrics,
Cambridge Hospital and Mt. Auburn Hospital,
Cambridge, Massachusetts

Virginia S. Villani, M.D.
Former Director, Bay Cove Day Center for Children,
New England Medical Center Hospitals,
Boston, Massachusetts

Preface

The knowledge and skills required in the clinical practice of child psychiatry have burgeoned rapidly over the past 25 years. The breadth and pace of these changes confront both child fellows and practitioners with a vast number of learning tasks related to a variety of disciplines: clinical medicine, psychopharmacology, genetics, education, and the law. As a result, the "classical" clinical models—based primarily on development and psychoanalysis—no longer suffice to integrate current clinical essentials; the "glue" sometimes is missing and ambiguity becomes the rule. The biopsychosocial approach to clinical data gathering and the resurgence of the "medical model" show promise as foundations of clear clinical thinking. These foundations are capable, in general, of incorporating both old and new knowledge and skills. Such a point of view is reflected in this manual.

Although there are many general and specialized textbooks in child psychiatry, a concise, practical but comprehensive guidebook to clinical practice is a timely project. This volume is designed as a working manual for fellows in child psychiatry. It should guide them through the basic, practical tasks of residency training. However, medical students, residents in general psychiatry, pediatricians, family practitioners, and other child mental health professionals should find the book useful. By distilling, condensing, and summarizing fundamental knowledge and skills, this manual can function as a basis for

---

I would like to thank Bonnie D. Cummins, M.Ed., for her excellent editorial assistance and Patricia A. McNamara for her help in typing the manuscripts. Mrs. John Duggan's assistance in many aspects of this book are especially appreciated.

the development of sound, competent, and broadly based clinical expertise.

Central to the overall purpose of the manual is to gather together, in one relatively small volume, essential clinical materials that currently are scattered throughout a vast number of journals, books, and texts. To fulfill this purpose, the format is designed to orient the reader to basic principles rather than detailed "fine tuning." In general, to maintain a book of convenient size, clinical examples have been left to a minimum throughout the text. Parts 1 and 2 present thorough coverage of diagnostic and therapeutic issues. Consultation and some related clinical issues reviewed in Part 3 have been selected to address certain "high incidence" areas of contemporary clinical concern for which rapidly available, practical guidance is unavailable. This last section is not, therefore, intended to be comprehensive. However, these special topics tend to relate to the consultative role of the child psychiatrist in areas of increasing clinical importance.

The chapters are organized around the traditional medical examination. Although *DSM-III* poses problems, it is used in relation to diagnostic considerations throughout the text. Because this volume is not a comprehensive text, brief, germane bibliographies appear at the end of each chapter.

The editor and most contributors are affiliated with the Division of Child Psychiatry, New England Medical Center Hospitals/Tufts University School of Medicine. Past and present staff members and child fellows within this program are represented. I am grateful for the contributors' participation in this book and for the opportunity of working with them over the past decade.

This book is dedicated to Arthur Z. Mutter, M.D., Chief of the Division of Child Psychiatry. He is a colleague, friend, and teacher, and the architect of the clinical services that made this volume possible.

Kenneth S. Robson, M.D.

PART 1
DIAGNOSTIC ASSESSMENT

Chapter 1.	Introduction to Diagnostic Assessment	3
Chapter 2.	Diagnostic Assessment: Technical Considerations	21
Chapter 3.	Physical and Neurological Examinations and Laboratory Studies	35
Chapter 4.	Psychological Testing	65
Chapter 5.	Formulation, Differential Diagnosis, and Treatment Planning	103

Chapter 1

Introduction to Diagnostic Assessment

Kenneth S. Robson, M.D.

THE NATURE OF CHILDHOOD PSYCHOPATHOLOGY

In approaching the diagnostic process in child psychiatry, the relationships among developmental phenomena, psychopathology and systems of classification (nosology) are frequently confused (1). Furthermore, the models underlying these three clinical arenas are blurred by the patchwork utilization of terms, concepts, and schools of thought that obscures clarity of thinking.

To begin, normative development and mental health are synonymous in childhood. Development may be defined as a progressive process resulting from the interplay between biological maturation and environmental influences. Growth, consolidation of functions, mastery, and integration—all aspects of development—are the central core of healthy functioning in childhood. Conversely, all forms of psychopathology in childhood and adolescence involve varying degrees of developmental deviance. Whether catastrophic and relatively fixed as in autism and childhood schizophrenia, or minimal and transient as in the adjustment disorders of the preschool child, these developmental deviations result from some combination of biological, psychological, and sociocultural factors. The goal of the diagnostic process is to identify these pathogenic factors clearly, particularly those subject to some form of modification. The aim of all therapeutic interventions is to eliminate or alter these "pathogens" in order to facilitate development.

Models of development in the child psychiatric literature are offered by seminal theorists such as Sigmund Freud, Anna Freud, Melanie Klein, Erik Erikson, Donald Winnicott, Heinz Werner, Jean Piaget, Heinz Kohut, Margaret Mahler, and Robert White (2). Each of these authors and others have made significant contributions to particular areas of development, or particular points of view across the continuum of the life cycle. A distillate of Erikson's epigenetic cycle and stages of development (3) and Anna Freud's concepts of developmental lines (4) provides a useful template of development against which to view the disturbances of childhood and adolescence.

Erikson conceived of development as a series of specific tasks generally conforming to more or less discrete ages in childhood and adolescence. Failures in one stage of development leave "unfinished business" for subsequent stages. For example, an infant who fails to establish "basic trust" during the first year of life will be plagued by distrust in later relationships. Erikson's model is cross-sectional and assumes, in general, that all aspects of development are delayed or advanced in unison. Anna Freud, on the other hand, elaborated a series of longitudinal developmental lines or systems that, while closely related to one another, may and often do proceed at different rates in relation to chronological age, developmental interferences, and pathogenic conditions. These lines include cognition and interpersonal relations. Indeed, it is clinically true that children referred for psychiatric evaluation exhibit differential progress in certain lines of development. The 5-year-old with precocious speech who is encopretic illustrates the usefulness of this model.

If one loosely combines the cross-sectional and longitudinal concepts of Erikson and A. Freud, the result is a kind of "exoskeleton" of development that seems to be a useful vehicle for clinical thinking and the integration of other developmental issues, lines, and systems. This perspective is illustrated in Figure 1. Within this diagram the cross-sectional phases/tasks of Erikson are supported by the developmental lines of Anna Freud. Both models relate to one another but view the process of development from differing perspectives. Such an ideogram also permits the student of child psychiatry to insert and incorporate particular authors (e.g., Klein, Winnicott, and Mahler) and subsystems of development (e.g., CNS maturation, affect tolerance) into one construct.

The relationship of development to pathology is complex and sometimes confusing. At times developmental deviance itself, particularly in the less serious disorders seen in preschoolers (e.g., reactions to stress, transient sleep, toileting, and behavioral disturbances) represent "pathology" without intrinsic disease process. Other conditions such as Tourette's disease, autism, and schizophrenia more closely approximate the traditional medical model of illness; massive and persistent developmental arrests are always present. In these latter disorders the pathologic process seems to have its own line of development that weaves its way, like a vine, into the interstices of normal developmental potential, eroding and stifling as it grows. In still other syndromes, such as attention deficit disorders (ADD), the teasing out of developmental issues as apart from pathologic process may be evident only with the passage of time. Some children with ADD at age 5 or 6 may be asymptomatic in all respects by adolescence; others progress into borderline states or frank psychosis in puberty. But again, *all* childhood disorders are either defined or accompanied by some developmental skewing.

Normal developmental progress requires optimal and sensitively modulated levels of internal and external stimulation delivered by an empathic, nonintrusive, and respectful caretaking environment. In general, every child referred for psychiatric evaluation or treatment suffers from excessively intense internal and external stimulation and some degree of empathic failure in the caretaking environment. Excessive stimulation may arise from too much or too little excitement or arousal, or as is more usual in clinical practice, both. The functional

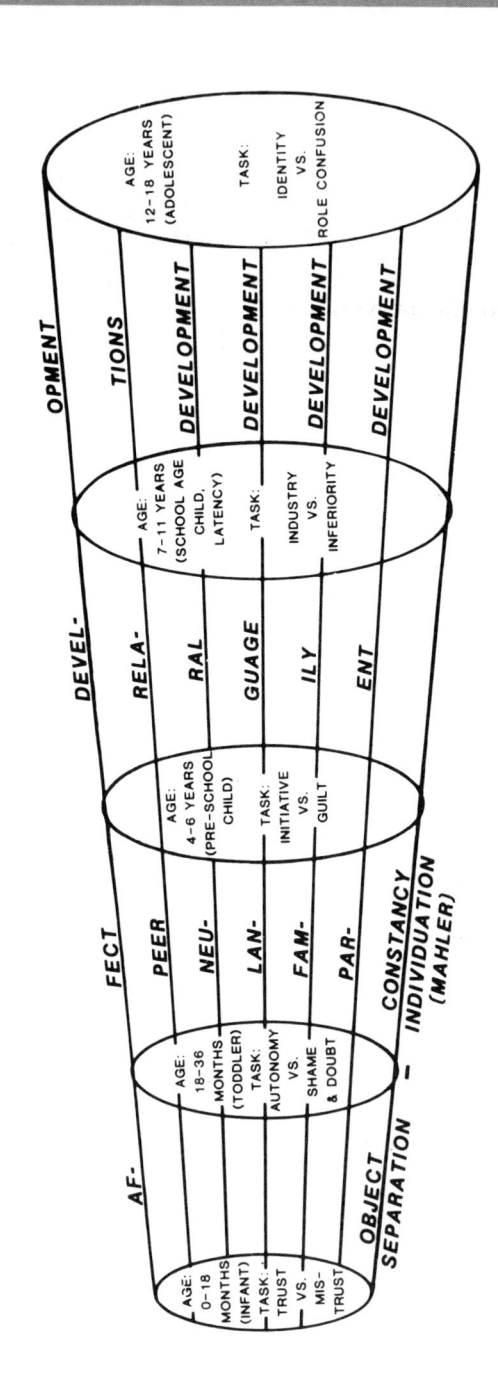

Figure 1. "Exoskeleton" Model of Development Combining the Cross-Sectional and Longitudinal Concepts of Erikson and A. Freud

result within the child is the same: *flooding* of the child's ego so as to interfere with or prohibit developmental processes. The brain-damaged or constitutionally hypersensitive child, for example, is easily stressed or disorganized by normal levels of environmental noise, physical handling, or the internal stimulation of puberty. On the other hand, parental overstimulation, whether seductiveness and physical excess or neglect and abrupt withdrawal, so floods the inner world of the child that various patterns of developmental deviance are inevitable. These include poor separation-individuation, cognitive disruption, impulse control problems, and more grave disturbances.

From his vast clinical experience, Donald Winnicott (5) describes two fundamental modes of relatedness that respectively interfere with or enhance development. The "orgiastic" mode is characterized by poor respect for interpersonal boundaries, peaks and valleys of stimulation and contact, and recurrent flooding of the developing child's ego. The "ego-relatedness" mode is an opposite mode that empathically modulates stimulation levels, observes interpersonal separateness, and creates the quiet space so essential for the crystals of development to take their shape. Within the schema being described here, the orgiastic mode is to some extent present in all forms of childhood psychopathology and ego-relatedness to some extent the therapeutic goal. Adult manifestations of overstimulation and empathic failure are manifest in such problems as "intensity," poor impulse control; lability of self-esteem, affects, and relationships; and narcissistic concerns.

This manner of describing and understanding psychopathology does not eliminate the need for precise understanding of pathologic phenomena of every variety (e.g., neurologic, biochemical, perceptual, cognitive, and interpersonal). Nor does it bypass rigorous differential diagnoses and the use of the *Diagnostic and Statistical Manual of Mental Disorders, Third Edition (DSM-III)* (6). Rather, it weaves such data together as they affect the envelope of internal and external "atmospheric" conditions surrounding the child. Empathic caretaking and modulated levels of stimulation are the critical clinical principles, the "thermostats," by which the child psychiatrist gains understanding of the broad picture of psychopathology, designs therapeutic interventions, and assesses their success. This perspective of development and childhood psychopathology views internal or external conflict as relatively unimportant in causing pathologic states. In most instances a child's conflicts such as those over the expression of aggression or "oedipal concerns" will resolve themselves in the context of empathic parenting and appropriately modulated levels of stimulation. The clinical usefulness of this point of view will be discussed in subsequent sections of this manual. Some aspects of this perspective on childhood psychopathology are summarized in Figure 2.

Within Figure 2 examples of external overstimulation and empathic failure coexist, as is the case in clinical practice. Indeed, overstimulation is always associated with empathic failure. In the therapeutic side of clinical practice, one addresses one or both problems in relation to such considerations as timing, stability, and depth of the therapeutic alliance with parents. In general, environmental overstimulation and empathic failures contribute to the larger variance in their effects on developing psychopathology.

THE MEDICAL MODEL IN CHILD PSYCHIATRIC DIAGNOSIS

Like the history of child psychiatry itself, the diagnostic process involved in the clinical appraisal of childhood disorders involves data from several disciplines, including pediatrics, psychoanalysis, education, social work, clinical child psychology, and child development (7). Not surprisingly, a multiplicity of philosophies, systems, and nosologies have emerged to cover and confuse the diagnostic landscape. The dominant role of clinical medicine and its models in American child psychiatry is a recent trend. As a result, the beginning clinician, usually trained in general psychiatry as well as other medical specialties, is often anxious and confused about both where and how to begin. Furthermore, the knowledge and skills of experienced nonphysician colleagues (e.g., social

Figure 2. The Pathophysiology of Childhood Disorders

OVERSTIMULATION		EMPATHIC FAILURES
INTERNAL (CHILD)	EXTERNAL (PARENTS)	
"Hyperacusis" to sound, talk, etc.	Seductive & erotizing physical contact & closeness	Misunderstanding of child's behavior
CNS hypersensitivity (second degree) to brain damage	Abrupt withdrawal in anger	Difficulty in accurately identifying child's inner states
Impulsivity	Emotional unavailability (as in depression or schizoid states)	"Spoiling"
Erotization of physical contact	Frightening behavior (physical or emotional)	Misperception of child's capacities in reaction to age
Intolerance of affects	Open bathroom doors	Misreading child's needs
Rejection sensitivity	Persistent and inappropriate teasing	Difficulty in treating child as separate person (i.e., treating child as "self-object")
Panic anxiety	Child sleeping in parent bed	Need for child as sustaining object
Poorly regulated and labile self-esteem	Extreme & age-inappropriate expectations	Rigid replaying of one's own parents unempathic caretaking
Rigid ego ideal	"Intrusiveness" and lack of respect for child's boundaries	"Identification with the aggressor"
Overly harsh conscience	Physical and sexual abuse	
Impatience and inability to delay gratification of wishes	Open bedroom doors	
Narcissistic entitlement	Communal toileting and bathing	

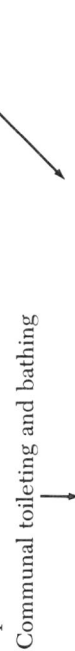

DEVELOPMENTAL DEVIANCE IN SPECIFIC PATHOLOGIC STATES

workers, child care staff, clinical psychologists) may threaten the sense of "seniority" and clinical competence established in the general residency before starting child psychiatric training. In addition, to play with children as an essential part of one's medical work can seem initially incongruous or even alarming. Such concerns in the entry level child fellow are to some extent inevitable, generally short-lived, and a part of the identity reorganization that accompanies the acquisition of new skills. It is useful to keep in mind that the psychiatrist completing both general and child residency training is the true physician "generalist" in the field. One of the particular pleasures of the specialty is the capacity to exercise psychiatric skills across the entire life cycle in relation to individual children, adolescents, adults, parents, marital couples, and families.

A clear conception of the systems of classification underlying child psychiatric diagnostic work guides learning and reduces ambiguity. The data relevant to any clinical syndrome or entity are best gathered from the biopsychosocial "pool." The interaction of biological, psychological, and social variables in the etiologies of pathological conditions in childhood, although not always obvious, is consistently true. Furthermore, although not all child psychiatric diagnoses are readily classified as disease entities, the traditional medical model is sufficiently broad to integrate all varieties of childhood psychopathology. The use of this model is also consistent with the diagnostic classification of *DSM-III*. The organization of clinical data within the standard medical case history described in this chapter encourages clear and rigorous diagnostic thinking, sound treatment planning, well-executed write-ups, authoritative case presentations, and effective communication with medical colleagues. In diagnosing childhood psychopathology, the use of biopsychosocial perspective focused through the lens of the medical model and *DSM-III* is strongly recommended.

THE CASE HISTORY

The data base gathered in child psychiatric diagnosis is substantially larger than in general psychiatry. Because the child patient can provide only limited information, the child psychiatrist must turn to others (i.e., parents, teachers, agency staff, medical colleagues). Furthermore, because assessments of current life functioning are so essential for both diagnostic process and treatment planning, in-depth data from the child's family and institutional affiliations (e.g., schools, foster homes, therapeutic settings, courts) are required. Assembling these data in a concise and logical format, however, is difficult. Furthermore, in time one learns that certain data are irrelevant in most instances. Careful, tactful working on the clinician's part is necessary to elicit data from expectably defensive parents. A diagnostic template such as that described below is extraordinarily valuable to the beginning clinician; it provides a kind of clinical road map to the diagnostic process. The case history that follows has proven useful to child fellows, general residents, medical students, and other professional trainees. The order in which data are organized and presented in this schema is designed to maximize clear diagnostic thinking; this order should be maintained. For example, the elaboration of the family history before developmental history places the latter immediately in the context of the child's world. Because divisions of child psychiatry frequently utilize many forms for recording diagnostic data, this case history can be modified when necessary. As a tool this format is especially helpful in determining which data to gather; organizing those data; developing differential diagnostic thinking; facilitating treatment planning; and communicating results clearly to parents, colleagues, courts, schools, and so on, and within teaching settings.

CHILD PSYCHIATRIC CASE HISTORY/DIAGNOSTIC FORMAT

With experience the clinician soon learns shortcuts to the most valuable data, particularly in the early stages of a diagnostic work-up when decisions regarding treatment and hospitalization must be made.

Chief Complaint/Presenting Problem

A few sentences concisely summarizing the primary reason and source of the referral. Include child's name, parent's/family's name, sex, age, race, religion, and birth order. The precise reasons for the referral—in the words of the referral source—should be used whenever possible. If this is not the first referral to the service, that fact should be noted.

Present Illness/Precipitating Stress

A brief description of the interpersonal, intrapsychic, and environmental circumstances leading up the development of the chief complaint/presenting problem and referral. This section of the work-up is obviously more relevant to situations with an *acute* onset and should include illness, loss of a family member, moves, and developmental changes (e.g., weaning, menarche). The *absence* of precipitating stresses is significant and should be noted.

Family History, Family Composition, and Home Environment

A concise but thorough description beginning with the current family composition and including three generations. A family tree offers a rapid visual presentation of complicated data (Figure 3).

The data base should include names, birth dates, parental marital history, dates of separations, hospitalizations, divorces, deaths, abortions, and stillbirths; specify both month and year of these events. Family history of medical conditions, major mental illness, "nervous breakdowns," tics, alcoholism, drug addiction, seizures, and mental retardation should be noted. These data can be appended to the family tree and are helpful in establishing any possible genetic base for a psychiatric illness. In addition, brief summaries of each parent's life events should be added and events pertaining to their own development emphasized.

A description of the house or apartment—including neigh-

Introduction to Diagnostic Assessment 13

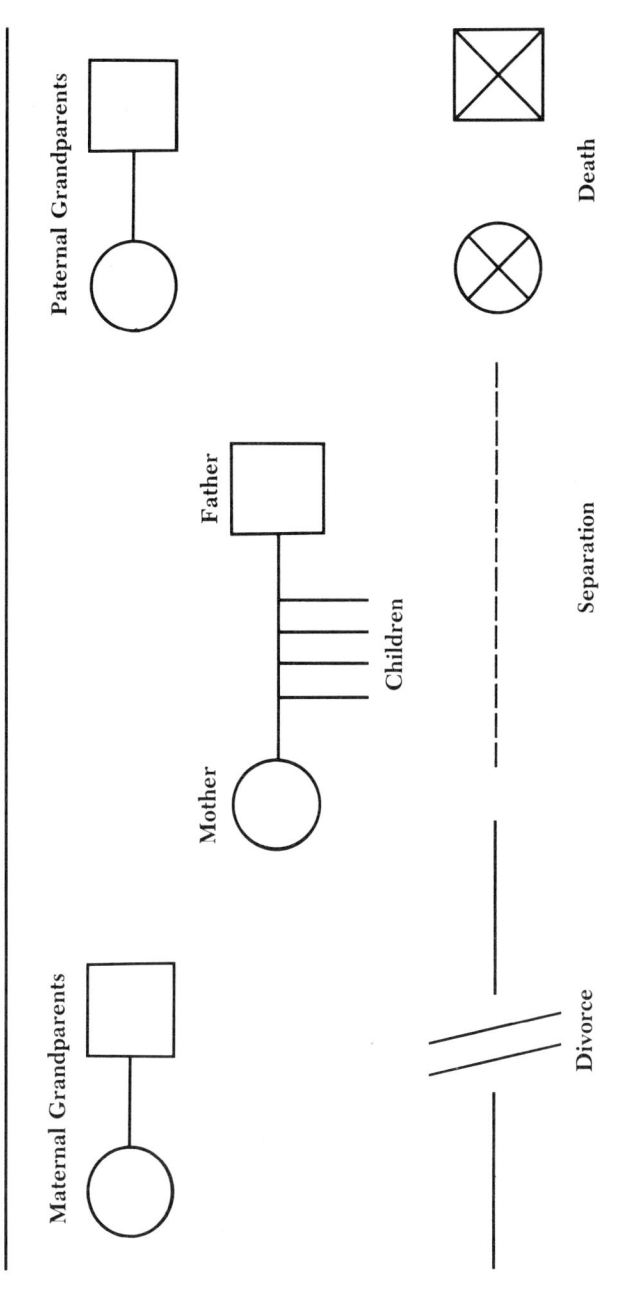

Figure 3. Descriptive Symbols Used in Composing a Family Tree

borhood, number of rooms and floors, location of child's and parents' rooms, sibling's rooms, and bathrooms—should be gathered. Toileting and bathing style and customs (e.g., bathroom doors open, nudity, bathing together) can be noted.

DEVELOPMENTAL HISTORY

Pregnancy. Parity and gravid status of mother at time of conception, medical complications, weight gain/loss, attitudes of parent(s) toward pregnancy, well-being of mother, any complicating life events, preference for girl or boy.

Labor and delivery. Medical complications (e.g., fetal distress, jaundice), birth weight, Apgar scores if available (request birth records if any question about complications or prematurity), mother's feelings surrounding her impression of baby (e.g., family resemblance, personality characteristics), choice of baby's name, maternal depression, anergy.

Infancy (0–18 mo). Medical problems first 18 months, feeding patterns, irritability, sleeping patterns, rocking and head banging, onset and intensity of stranger anxiety (being strange with people) and separation protest behavior, unusual fearfulness and unusual sensitivity to loud noises (e.g., blender, vacuum cleaner, sirens, unfamiliar settings), indiscriminate response to others, "cuddliness" with mother and others, onset and nature of speech (*crucial*), gross motor milestones (e.g., sitting, walking), prolonged separations and parental illness.

Toddler (18–36 mo). Onset and success of toilet training; presence and nature of externally directed aggression including temper tantrums, fears, and night terrors; socialization; separation behavior; sleeping patterns and whether child sleeps in parental bed (and frequency); speech development; development of autonomy and self-control; contest "struggles."

Preschool (4–6 yr). Socialization, adjustment to nursery school and kindergarten, peer relations, fears, impulse control, curiosity, assertiveness, soiling/smearing, enuresis, management of aggression, masturbation, coordination, clumsiness, nightmares, whether child sleeps in parental bed (and frequency).

Latency (6–11 yr). Peer relations (e.g., best friends), interests, hobbies, sports, cognitive gains, impulse control, coordination, clumsiness, separations (e.g., camp), and reactions to them.

Puberty and adolescence (12–16 yr). Secondary sexual characteristics, masturbation, menarche, alcohol, tobacco, drugs, regressions in learning and/or behavior, depression, withdrawal, peer relations.

School History

Current school. Name and address of school, grade, names of teachers (homeroom, guidance counselor, principal), grades (request report cards) and any changes within the past year in grades and/or behavior in school. If involved in present or past special education program, obtain summaries.

Past school history. Adjustment to first school experience, separation problems, school refusal ("phobia"), behavior problems, failing or acceleration.

Medical History

Date, place, and physician carrying out most recent physical examination and results; all significant illnesses, operations, and injuries since birth with dates, hospital(s), and outcome; history of allergies and current use of medications.

Interviews with Child and Mental Status Examination

A concise but thorough description of observations during interviews. Include general appearance and behavior, relatedness, dominant mood/affect, coordination and movement, speech and language, perception/cognition, play, conscience/impulse control, self-concept (see Chapter 2). For practical purposes in write-ups or presentations, a summary of those aspects of the mental status examination and interview content is essential for differential diagnosis and disposition.

Interviews with Family

Description of family. Members present, number and dates of interviews.

Summary of interviews. Seating arrangement(s) (draw), quality of interactions, key reactors, major themes, quality of communication, ability to listen to one another, respect for separateness, prevailing mood and affect, degree of concern for one another, "enmeshment/disengagement," family's view of child's problem (will family support or resist therapy of child), manner in which family has managed child's problem to date.

Auxiliary Data

Psychological testing, neurological evaluations, laboratory data.

Formulation

A brief but salient synthesis of all previous biopsychosocial data, the intent of which is to convey the chronological internal and external event-related development of the child's problem. This summary, a critical portion of the work-up, should include biogenetic factors; primary conflict(s); psychosexual level of development (see, Freud, Erikson); primary defenses utilized ("ego strength"); degree that problem is ego-syntonic or ego-alien, internalized, acute or chronic.

The formulation should include relevant family data such as stage of family development (7); style of family functioning (8,9); family defenses, preoccupations, losses, and shifts; and quality of object relations. Identification and listing of primary problem facilitates treatment planning.

Diagnosis

The diagnostic considerations should flow naturally from the formulation and conform to that data base. Differential diagnoses should be listed and a working final diagnosis noted in relation to *DSM-III*.

Plan

This is a brief description of the therapeutic plan, including psychotherapy, medication, school modification, and environmental manipulations.

FURNISHING THE OFFICE PLAYROOM

The psychiatric assessment of a child can be conducted in virtually any setting. Whether schoolroom, hospital bedside, the child's own home, or the office playroom, the critical variables are the comfort of the examiner and the quality of contact with the child. Valuable diagnostic data can be gathered rapidly and accurately by the physician who can and should relax, enjoy, and explore the clinical process spontaneously. Hence, in most respects, the attitudes and behaviors of the diagnostician are the most important "furnishings" in successful clinical work. Nonetheless, the office playroom is a major workspace and deserves attention.

In some clinical settings, office and playroom are separate from one another. Although some clinicians prefer such an arrangement, it is by no means necessary. The combined space has the advantage of flexibly encouraging play and/or verbal interchange for children of all ages. Such an arrangement is useful in family meetings where both "adult" and "child" space is required. In addition to adult-size desk and chairs, a smaller table and chairs to match for younger children is helpful. Personal and homey touches, such as an electric water heater for instant coffee, cocoa, and soup and a jar or box with crackers or nuts, create a pleasant atmosphere, are useful diagnostic tools in their own right, and facilitate alliance formation with both children and parents. Hospitality and informality need not be incompatible with professional competence. A cup of coffee for an anxious parent can establish a sense of safety and comfort that is work-enhancing. Photographs of the diagnostician's spouse and children probably do *not* belong in the office playroom.

A bulletin board is almost essential for children's drawings. A calendar and maps of the local city, state, and country are useful diagnostic and therapeutic aids. Space to keep the projects and products of children in therapy may be located in the examiner's desk or on a shelf. Shoe boxes can serve the same purpose and, when identified by the child's name, can lend privacy and continuity to clinical work.

Obviously some collection of toys and games is important. The beginning clinician is well-guided by the principle that "less is more." Most children brought to the child psychiatrist suffer from some form of overstimulation (particularly in the American culture). Too many bright, novel, and interesting objects often lead to chaos, overactivity, and a nervous and harried examiner. *The most valuable diagnostic tool is one's self.* Material objects, especially in excess, complicate and confuse the diagnostic process. Furthermore, the uses and limitations of various play objects should be kept in mind. They are not present to entertain or distract (either examiner or child); their primary purposes are, in order of importance:

- To serve as a medium for contact/relatedness with the child;
- To inform the diagnostician about cognitive, affective, and perceptual capacities or deficits; and
- To facilitate developmental progress in therapies.

At the same time, selecting items that are of interest to or skill areas of the examiner is perfectly reasonable as long as they are not used to protect his or her own sense of competence against the natural anxieties of beginning clinical work with children.

Some practical items from which to make selections, by age, are as follows:

Infant/Toddler (1–3 yr). One or two dolls, large rubber or Nerf® ball, pull or push toy such as large wooden train with cars that connect.

Preschooler (4–6 yr). Drawing and construction materials (crayons, felt-tip markers, paper, scissors, stapler, paste, and adhesive tape), doll house, hand and finger puppets, family figurines, anatomically correct dolls, toy guns, toy soldiers, Lincoln Logs® or Tinker Toys®, Matchbox® cars, simple card games (e.g., fish, war, old maid) on large decks with pictures, simple board games (e.g., Candyland®, Chutes and Ladders®), books, Play-Doh®, old newspapers, water paints.

School Age (7–12 yr). Books, deck of cards, Nerf® basketball set, soft rubber dart gun, Velcro® darts and target, games (e.g., chess, checkers, Othello®, Score Four®, dominoes, Labyrinth®, table top sports games, model building equipment (pen knife with retractable blade, Duco® cement, cutting board), cassettes for tape recording stories and play.

Some of these items are useful starters. All may be used by any age group (including adolescents), depending on the level of development or the phase of treatment or play therapy. Whenever possible, it is best to keep one's play equipment behind shelf doors to avoid overstimulation. The examiner needs to encourage spontaneity and to maintain control.

REFERENCES

1. Shapiro T: The borderline syndrome in children: a critique, in The Borderline Child. Edited by Robson K. New York, McGraw-Hill, 1983

2. Bemporad J: Child Development in Normality and Psychopathology. New York, Brunner/Maxel, 1980
3. Erikson EH: Childhood and Society. New York, Norton, 1963
4. Freud A: The concept of developmental lines. Psychoanal Study Child 18:245–265, 1963
5. Winnicott DW: The location of cultural experience. Int J Psychoanal 48:368–372, 1967
6. American Psychiatric Association: Diagnostic and Statistical Manual of Mental Disorders, Third Edition. Washington, DC, American Psychiatric Association, 1980
7. Group for the Advancement of Psychiatry: Psychopathological Disorders in Childhood: Theoretical Considerations and a Proposed Classification. New York, Group for the Advancement of Psychiatry, 1966
8. Zilbach J: Family development, in Basic Handbook of Child Psychiatry. Edited by Noshpitz J. New York, Basic Books, 1979
9. Minuchin S: Families and Family Therapy. Cambridge, Harvard University Press, 1974
10. Skynner ACR: Systems of Family and Marital Psychotherapy. New York, Brunner/Mazel, 1976

Chapter 2

Diagnostic Assessment: Technical Considerations

Kenneth S. Robson, M.D.

GOALS OF THE DIAGNOSTIC PROCESS

In child psychiatry, less is often more in all aspects of clinical work. The natural force and momentum of growth and development are powerful allies to the clinician and increase the likelihood of modest change leading to significant therapeutic results. Skillful management of diagnostic assessments can prove to be substantial interventions in the life of a child. Thus, even more than in general psychiatry, the alert diagnostician needs to couple a therapeutic stance with clear but flexible goals in the evaluation of children. These goals tend to separate into first and second stage issues:

First Stage Diagnostic Issues

- To establish whether emergency intervention is required (see Chapter 10).
- To develop positive contact with the referral source.
- To explore financial issues sufficiently to consider their relevance in the evaluation (see "Parent Interviews" below).

- To decide who should be involved in the initial clinical session.
- To gather as much clinical data as necessary from the family, child, and other agencies to reach a preliminary diagnosis sufficient to make decisions regarding a working plan of treatment; extended diagnostic evaluations; or referral elsewhere. Decisions to treat or refer are often possible long before comprehensive diagnostic data are available or necessary.

Second Stage Issues

- To refine and elaborate preliminary diagnostic impressions via clinical contacts, psychological testing, laboratory tests, and school consultation.
- To define the developmental needs and deficits of the child clearly (i.e., separation from parents, establishment of autonomy, enhancement of peer relations, and the means to address them).
- To integrate all existing data into a comprehensive treatment plan. Given the nature of child psychiatry, such treatment planning is complex and resembles good choreography—timing is critical! For example, a child's need for intensive psychotherapy, a therapeutic school, or psychoactive medication may be quickly evident to the clinician but not recommended until parental support for such steps is established.

THE CLINICAL APPROACH IN CHILD PSYCHIATRY

The resident in general psychiatry, and in other medical specialties, learns a professional bearing with patients and families that may encourage formality and relative distance. In child psychiatry, such a bearing may complicate work with children and parents. A comfortable but appropriate informality is likely to be more effective. Pleasantness, small talk and chattiness, and *active* efforts to help new and always anxious patients feel at ease are compatible with excellent care. For example, offering parents coffee or soup on a cold day can accelerate alliance formation and the diagnostic process. Further, one's own personality, life experiences, memories, interests, and beliefs are valuable assets to be thoughtfully, professionally, and comfortably *used* rather than obscured. Being "one's self" is not unprofessional. The child psychiatrist's capacity to play and enjoy it *belong* in the clinical process. A few points:

- Parents are not patients. They are parents and should be treated as respected collaborators.
- Children like to know, and usually assume, that the doctor knows something about their world in the small ways that matter. Take every chance to reacquaint oneself with the activities, life space, and mundane details of children of all ages (e.g., current sports heroes, TV programs, breakfast cereals, movies, slang, drug names, shoe brands).
- Children are not little adults. Those who can relate like adults (i.e., sitting and talking) often don't need to.
- Reacquaint oneself with one's own childhood memories. Although at times painful, this is extraordinarily useful in developing empathy and clinical skills. Children often believe that adults cannot understand them and were never children themselves.
- Enjoy the work and expect anxiety, confusion, and occasional embarrassment as natural and temporary aspects of the job.

REFERRAL OF CHILDREN

Unlike adults, children, even most adolescents, rarely refer themselves for psychiatric care. They are in some sense captives of the family, foster care, or institution serving them in loco parentis. Further, the resistances to referral, particularly in biological families, are probably more powerful than is the case with individual adult patients. The child is enmeshed in a complex network of relationships in which a change may be perceived as threatening to an entire family system. In the normal course of events, growth and development impose a *loss* upon parents that is always difficult. In pathological situations, where children often serve as inappropriate but sustaining figures for a parent, the potential, and usually unconscious, threat of separation may color the referral process with danger. In addition, the inevitable, intense feelings of guilt and failure on the part of parents create further encumbrances to successful referral. For these reasons, the clinician's first and most essential task in the diagnostic process is to establish a sympathetic, empathic, nonjudgmental, and supportive stance with the family member making the referral. An early assessment of the "power structure" affecting the child's life is always useful and sometimes necessary. For example, a father who must pay the bills may need contact with the diagnostician if the referral is to succeed.

Because of the resistances to referral in biological families, most initial contacts or referral suggestions are made by other people involved in the child's life. In order of usual frequency these include: teachers/schools; social service agencies; courts; and pediatricians, family practitioners, and other mental health professionals. Sensitivity to the needs and feelings of these referral sources is equally important. Prompt return of telephone calls and letters of acknowledgment, progress, and planning should be habitual.

There are often many "hidden agendas" in referrals of children. This is particularly true when multiple referral sources are involved (e.g., school and parents, or agency and parents). As noted above, the politics of referrals are often complex. In relation to the question of who should be seen first—child, parents, family, or referral source—it is generally useful to retain flexibility. The clinician usually can establish the most critical party with whom to initiate contact in the first meeting. Parents may need to "check out" the clinician first. Perhaps the child, as repository of all family psychopathology, can serve as the only acceptable entry point. Such needs must be understood and respected. In rare instances parents may insist, generally defensively, that the child be seen first because the child is "the patient." If that is not the case, with preadolescent children it is helpful in an initial visit to see the parents alone briefly to establish contact, then the family together, and then to spend some time alone with the child before his or her next visit. Adolescents more often are seen alone initially, although "enmeshed" families may require a group session or sessions in some instances. Premature insistence on a rigid diagnostic format may lose the referral. The beginning clinician will profit from exploring a variety of formats with the collaboration of an experienced clinician.

THE CLINICAL DIAGNOSTIC INTERVIEWS

"Agency" Referrals

In clinic settings, and increasingly in private practice, children are referred by courts, lawyers, special educators, and agency staff in state welfare offices. Such referrals are complex, often involving adversarial and fiscal issues between agencies and biological or foster families with conflicting ideas about the child's best interest. Questions of custody, abuse, and "fitness" are common. Support for a special educational placement may be deemed too costly and unnecessary. The clinician who accepts such a referral without first clarifying the issues may waste extraordinary amounts of time while limiting the usefulness of the assessment. In situations of this kind, it is wise to establish *beforehand*:

- Who are all of the interested parties, what are their respective roles in the child's life, and "who wants what from whom"?
- What are the limits and characteristics of your role in the evaluation (e.g., clinical evaluator, consultant, potential expert witness)? To whom will you have access? The diagnostician needs maximal leeway and data and may wish to see biological parents and foster parents, for example. In general, the safest and most important role for the child psychiatrist is as evaluator of and advocate for the child involved.
- Is the case now in litigation or is that route anticipated? If so, will you be expected to testify? Can and should you?

- What financial arrangements are involved if court time is likely to occur?

Careful prior assessment of these issues, whether by telephone or in person, is the prerogative of the child psychiatrist. Numerous cases of this kind may not be appropriate referrals but are difficult to interrupt once initiated.

Parent Interviews

The decision to have one's child evaluated is difficult to reach and is fraught with anxiety for most parents who feel exposed, vulnerable, and certain of their presumed failure. To be sympathetic and empathetic but not prematurely reassuring is useful. Whenever possible it is wise to leave the details of an evaluation (e.g., precise number of sessions with parents and child) open. A general description of the format, however, is comforting. Mentioning that meeting with the entire family at some point in the diagnostic process would be helpful can facilitate that part of the evaluation. Ordinarily one or two meetings with a parent or parents, one or two meetings with the child, auxiliary data gathering when indicated (e.g., pyschological testing, laboratory tests), and a wrap-up session with parents (and sometimes the child) suffice to reach first stage decisions.

Financial questions often arise in an initial telephone contact. The influence of fiscal realities on clinician options and planning is increasingly powerful and is in many cases a limiting factor in accomplishing evaluations or treatment. For example, many third-party payers have annual maximums, particularly for outpatient work; to use up these monies in an extensive evaluation may deprive the child of treatment. Psychological testing may be delayed in many situations where its cost would compromise treatment options. A diagnostic hospitalization, generally considered in relation to questions of serious disturbance, may sometimes be justified on economic as well as clinical grounds because inpatient insurance coverage is usually more extensive. Finally, in many clinics and hospitals limits on "bad debt" and "free care" control levels of fee adjustments and length of stay. The diagnostician needs to be well informed about local fiscal regulations and relate them to initial planning with parents from the outset.

Another question facing the evaluator arises when the referred child is involved in a separated or divorced family. Generally, but not always, the custodial parent makes the first contact and probably should be seen alone first. Although the participation of the noncustodial or estranged parent may be essential, it is ordinarily wiser to meet the referring parent first. In such situations, however, the diagnostician may be told that the other parent has "no interest" in the child or the evaluation. Such is often far from the case and circumspection and patience are advised.

Assuming that parent(s) sessions have been scheduled, certain guidelines can be helpful. A semi-structured interview style is useful. Permitting parents to share their own perceptions of the child and their own anxieties can provide much useful data. Often specific details of developmental history are mentioned spontaneously and can be briefly explored without disrupting the spontaneous flow of material.

At some natural break point in the parent interviews, the gathering of specific developmental family history data is essential. Let the chief complaint guide and prioritize the areas to pursue. For example, where depressive concerns are part of a referral, a detailed family history of alcoholism and affective disease and the child's sleeping patterns are more imperative than neuromotor milestones or toilet training. Because the diagnostic process is frequently the beginning of treatment in many instances, the documentation of certain data can be delayed and treated as second stage phenomena.

It is of enormous practical significance to assess and document in a preliminary way, while gathering both family and developmental history, the levels of stimulation to which the child is exposed or responds (see Chapter 1). Questions such as whether the child sleeps in parental beds, bathes with parents, and likes physical contact are useful and nonthreatening. Are doors kept open or shut? Are transitions such as from home to school in the morning and bedtime at night calm and low intensity or abrupt and disruptive? Do mealtimes facilitate pleasant modulated contact among family members or does chaos and agitation prevail? These data can play a major role in increasing understanding and therapeutic leverage.

Given limited time, there are three functional areas of a child's life that provide enough data for first stage decisions regarding the degree of impairment and the need for therapeutic interventions: (a) school competence (work), (b) the presence and quality of peer relationships (love), and (c) level of personal distress (e.g., depression, anxiety) (play). Interviews that focus on these areas in sufficient detail are cost effective. Of course, there are situations where a child who functions well in these areas may need to be taken into treatment because of family dysfunction externalized onto a relatively healthy child.

Most parents will want to know about diagnosis and prognosis early in the evaluation, often before the child is seen. Premature reassurance and dire predictions should both be avoided.

If not brought up spontaneously, the question of what to tell the child about the evaluation is important to address. Parents can be told that evaluations do not damage children or create problems that were not there already. Children can be told directly that they are going to see a doctor who helps with worries and problems, identifying the specific issue with the child (e.g., school problems, depression, separation anxiety). Parents should be discouraged from lying to a child about the nature of the evaluation.

Increasing numbers of children are referred and brought to the diagnostician by persons in loco parentis such as foster parents, social workers affiliated with state agencies or institutions, child care staff, and lawyers. Data from such sources, and from schools and teachers as well, are obviously as critical as that from parents in intact families. The diagnostician may modify the principles and practices described above in such instances but the aims of the data gathering are, of course, the same.

Family Interviews

With the possible exception of those catastrophic conditions of childhood apparently dominated by biological determinants (e.g., autism, pervasive developmental disorders, Tourette's disease, major depression), the interpersonal environment of the child plays a dominant role in both hindering and facilitating developmental process. To see this environment in action during the diagnostic evaluation is, therefore, extraordinarily important. An observant clinician can note, in a single family session, crucial aspects of the child's world that can include:

- His or her role in the family (e.g., scapegoat, "pseudoparent" to a mother or father, lover).
- The quality of parental relatedness and the meaning of an absent parent or lost object.
- The mode of relating in the family as "enmeshment" or "disengagement" (1) and the primary family affect (2).
- Developmental arrests or pathology in other family members.
- Some sources of symptomatology in the child and, from these data, specific goals for subsequent therapeutic intervention.

Without being a family therapist, the diagnostician can relatively quickly learn to use "family work" in a flexible manner in both the evaluation and treatment of children. Further, the introduction of family sessions during the diagnostic phase can facilitate subsequent use of this approach in therapies that follow. A diagnostic family session is strongly recommended (3). Some principles to guide the clinician follow:

- Family sessions are stressful and extra efforts to put family members at ease should be made. The clinician must be active.
- Invite all members to attend and always include infants.
- Use a room large enough to accommodate adults and young children; the latter need space to move about, "peel off,"

and return to the central group. Some play materials such as crayons and paper should be readily available.
- Schedule 1¼ to 1½ hours for such sessions.
- Encourage communication but make it clear that no one has to talk about anything they would rather not. Similarly, forbid physical injury or destruction of property.
- The data from such meetings are vast. An observant clinician will not try to catch all interactions but rather the central issues of seating arrangements, dominant affect(s), and mode of relatedness. One will learn more by expecting less.

Child Interviews

For the beginning clinician, interviews with children are anxiety-provoking. The world of childhood, especially if one is not a parent, seems to be a foreign country. Further, the clinician must unlearn in many respects the posture assumed with adult patients who generally can talk and often observe themselves. Finally, the affects of children are intense and often quite uncomfortable to experience, including the reawakened traumas of one's own childhood years. Anxiety is to be expected.

Another source of confusion to the clinician is the presence of play as a communicative mode. When one is accustomed to following the complexities of adult thought and speech, play as a form of action (even more so when alternating with speech in the verbal child) is difficult to follow. A common error is to search for too much meaning in every sequence of play. Most play sequences derive from real-life experiences, not fantasies, and are better understood as communications about past or current realities. The best guide to the content of any child interview is the child's affect. Generally, if the clinician can gain a sense of the prevailing emotion (e.g., anxiety, terror, sadness, depression, anger, despair, agitation), play and other forms of communication fall readily into place and seem to make sense. To achieve this stance the main effort should be simply to join the child, be with him or her—that is at once the easiest and hardest of tasks. To strain at it, however, never works. To try for less in this regard is usually to gain more. The stories that children have to tell are basic ones—to listen is enough to know that they feel afraid, discouraged, mad, or unloved. One cannot diagnose a child without first establishing contact. Do not look for "mysteries." The central issues are generally self-evident.

It is important not to substitute toys, games, complicated psychological tests, or rigid interview techniques for spontaneous interchange with the child. A *few* pieces of age-appropriate play materials (see Chapter 1) will suffice to facilitate rapport. Selecting two or three age-appropriate play items before the interview provides an orientation for the child and reduces the likelihood of stimulus overload in both patient and diagnostician.

The more formal categories of data to be observed are as follows:

General Appearance and Behavior. Size, habitus, weight, coloring, gait, dress, grooming, facial expression, ease or difficulty coming with examiner and separating from parents, eyeglasses, physical defects, "oddness."

Relatedness. Style and quality of contact with the examiner, availability or genuineness of child, depth of contact, shallowness, precociousness, use of eye contact, seductiveness and excessive use or avoidance of physical contact, rate of relatedness (indiscriminate and immediate or avoidant and fearful). Change in depth of relatedness over time (within or across interviews) is especially important to note.

Dominant Mood/Affect. Depression (include suicidal ideation or plans), discouragement, apathy, anxiety, fear, panic, drivenness, anger, irritability; excitement, helplessness, optimism; blunting, shallowness, lability of affects.

Coordination and Movement. Clumsiness (examine for "soft" neurological signs, see Chapter 3), agility, level of activity, stiffness of bearing and gait, hand–eye coordination, abnormal involuntary movements including tics, tremors, choreo-athetosis, spasticity, and oral–buccal movement when evaluating for tardive dyskinesia. Minor physical anomalies may be noted (4).

Speech and Language. Vocabulary, expressive clarity, use in interpersonal communication; idiosyncrasies including punning, neologisms, echolalia, pronominal reversal; modulation of tone and intensity; paralinguistic richness versus "tin woodman" or metallic quality of speech; stuttering, complexity and age-appropriateness of verbal expressions; precocity of language.

Perception/Cognition. Integrity of vision and hearing; orientation to time, place, and person; confusion; attention and capacity to concentrate; level of intelligence and obvious learning impairments (capacity to read and do math problems can be examined); quality of thinking: logicality, organization, concreteness, ability to use symbolization and abstract thought, evidence of primary process; presence and durability of reality testing; content of thought: repetitive themes, preoccupation, richness, impoverishment, ability to fantasize at age-appropriate level; constriction or inhibition of thought.

Play. Spontaneity, choice of materials/activities, ability to involve examiner, capacity to sustain interest and elaborate themes, anxiety, and "play interruptions" (the abrupt cessation of a play sequence in relation to anxiety-provoking material); repetitive sequences.

Conscience/Impulse Control. Rigidity or laxity of conscience, stability of impulse control.

Self-Concept. Self-esteem, identifications, gender preference and perception. Asking a child to draw himself or herself is very helpful in this regard.

In time the beginning diagnostician will develop a style in conducting interviews with a child. In training it is especially useful to observe experienced clinicians interviewing one's patients; if not offered, it can be requested. In any event, the integration of these data may seem a staggering task. This task is simplified if one distills from the mental status examination its essential aims—namely, to become informed about (a) the overall integrity of the child's neuromotor and cognitive apparatus, (b) the child's capacity for relatedness, and (c) the status of his or her development vis-à-vis chronological age and the evenness or unevenness of major developmental "lines."

A general appreciation of each of these areas in conjunction with the stigmata of specific syndromes (e.g., the tics of Tourette's disease, vegetative signs of depression, thought disorder in schizophrenia) provides the diagnostician with ample information for the elaboration of differential diagnosis. However, data from the physical neurological examination, laboratory tests, and psychological assessments may also be necessary. Approaches to these data are described in Chapters 3 and 4. The integration of these data and their communication to others are discussed in Chapter 5.

References

1. Minuchin S: Families and Family Therapy. Cambridge, Harvard University Press, 1974

2. Fleck S: Family functioning and family pathology. Psychiatric Annals 10:17–35, 1980

3. Serrano AC: A child-centered family diagnostic interview, in Basic Handbook of Child Psychiatry. Edited by Noshpitz J. New York, Basic Books, 1980

4. Waldrop MF, Halverson CF: Minor physical anomalies and hyperactive behavior in young children, in Exceptional Infant, Vol. 2. Edited by Hellmuth J. New York, Brunner/Mazel, 1971

Chapter 3

Physical and Neurological Examinations and Laboratory Studies

P. S. B. Sarma, M.B., B.S.

William D. Singer, M.D.

Child psychiatric disorders are frequently associated with a number of medical findings in the physical appearance, physiological systems, and laboratory test data of the individual. These findings may simply accompany the psychiatric disorders without etiological significance. On the other hand, they may have more direct and significant relationships with psychiatric disorders in one or more of the following ways:

- Direct causal relationship (e.g., phenylketonuria and mental retardation).
- Indicator of deviation or insult at a specific point in development (e.g., first trimester related congenital anomalies).
- Indicator of predisposition to certain syndromes (e.g., low levels of dopamine B hydroxylase and certain conduct disorders).
- Indicator of recent insult to the nervous system (e.g., high lead levels in the blood).
- Probable indicator of prognosis (e.g., luteinizing hormone [LH] and follicle-stimulating hormone [FSH] patterns in clinically improved anorexia nervosa).

- Indicator of side effects from overzealous or even optimal treatment (e.g., electrocardiogram [EKG] changes associated with tricyclic antidepressant treatment).
- Features of the psychiatric disorders themselves (e.g., multiple superficial lacerations of the wrist in the histrionic and depressed adolescent girl or the low levels of growth hormone secretion seen in psychosocial dwarfism).

In the following pages the relevance of and indications for the use of established procedures will be discussed. Some new procedures that are helpful in the comprehensive psychiatric examination of children and adolescents will also be described.

THE PHYSICAL EXAMINATION

Most children and adolescents seen for evaluation in the office do not need to disrobe in order to undergo a rapid, selective physical examination. Five general indications for a complete physical examination include:

- *Major* psychiatric disturbances
- *Early onset* of the disturbance in the developmental spectrum
- Suspicion of *physical or sexual abuse* of the child
- *Substance abuse*
- Presenting problems that are clearly *physical* in nature (e.g., headaches, loss of weight)

Since every physician is trained to perform a physical examination, the details of this procedure will not be dealt with here. In the preschool age and in the early grade school age, it is advisable to record height and weight data routinely as well as the percentile scores. Heart rate and blood pressure should be recorded to compare against changes from the future treatments. Assessment of the integrity of the visual and auditory systems is especially important at all ages. These tests are generally performed in schools. However, if there is any doubt about the reliability of school reports, or if the reports are not available, it is advisable to use the Snellen charts for vision. Audiological screening is indicated for all children with problems in language skills, learning impairments, pervasive developmental disorders, and autism.

It is important that the child psychiatric physician be familiar with the dysmorphic features associated with the following conditions:

- Fetal alcohol syndrome, which can present with small head size, short palpebral fissures, drooping eyelids, epicanthal folds, maxillary hypoplasia, joint anomalies, cleft palate, capillary hemangioma, altered palmar creases, low birth weight, small-for-gestation size, a variety of cardiac anomalies, and significant delays in cognitive development.
- Fragile X syndrome, which can present with mental retardation, coarse facial features, large ears, prominent lower jaw, and large testicles.
- The various features associated with the long-recognized chromosomal anomalies such as Down's syndrome, Klinefelter syndrome, Turner syndrome, and those associated with tuberous sclerosis, neurofibromatosis, Prader-Willi syndrome, hypothyroidism, hyperthyroidism, and Lesch-Nyhan syndrome are important for the child psychiatrist to be aware of since the above conditions often have associated behavioral and/or cognitive deficits (see Chapter 16).

MINOR PHYSICAL ANOMALIES

In the last 10 years, minor physical anomalies (MPAs) have elicited increased attention not only in their relationships to the low incidence, high severity syndromes (e.g., autism), but also in their relationships to the high incidence, low severity types of behavioral disorders. MPAs indicate first trimester influences during intrauterine life and may be indicators of underlying neurological dysfunctions. Although hundreds of malformations related to the head, eyes, ears, hair, nose, mouth, palate, tongue, teeth, jaws, neck, extremities, digits, and body proportions are well catalogued by Smith (1), the studies conducted by Waldrop and Halverson (2) with a manageable number of MPAs are particularly useful to the psychiatrist. These authors reported significant correlations of high MPA scores with externalizing behaviors (hyperactivity and impulsivity) in boys and with fearful and inhibited behaviors in girls. These studies of MPAs are, unfortunately, confounded by inconsistent weights assigned to the different items. The neurological correlates of MPAs are not clearly established.

There are indications that in boys, MPAs correlate with high levels of serum dopamine-β-hydroxylase. This finding needs to be substantiated by other studies. MPAs continue to be a promising area for understanding the biological and genetic contributions to behavior. The MPAs studied by Waldrop and Halverson (2) are listed below. For excellent descriptions with illustrations, the reader is referred to their original report.

- Fine, electric hair
- Two or more hair whorls on the head
- Head circumference at least one standard deviation (SD) outside the normal range
- Epicanthic folds near the eyes
- Hyperteliorism
- Low-set ears
- Adherent ear lobes
- Malformed ears
- Asymmetrical ears
- Soft and pliable ears
- High-steepled palate
- Furrowed tongue
- Tongue with smooth-rough spots
- Curved fifth finger
- Single transverse palmar creases
- Third toe longer than second
- Partial syndactyly of two middle toes
- Big gap between first and second toes

NEUROLOGICAL EXAMINATION

It is clear that dysfunctions of the brain are related to significantly higher risk for psychiatric disorders in children (3). Hence, it is advisable that a psychiatric evaluation of the child utilize the "windows" that are available to assess brain function. The traditional neurological examination consisting of examination of the cranial nerves, motor strength, tone, coordination, speed, sensory integrity, deep tendon reflexes, and superficial reflexes has limited usefulness by itself for routine purposes. Obviously, children with localizing signs or neuropsychiatric syndromes will require a comprehensive examination by a pediatric neurologist (see Appendix 1 [4, 5]). Without specific indications, the use of some procedures such as neuropsychological batteries and the new generation of scan procedures—computed axial tomography (CAT), positron emission tomography (PET), nuclear magnetic resonance (NMR)—is neither clinically nor financially cost-effective. It is useful, however, to complete a brief, clinical office examination that will help select children for the more complex and expensive laboratory or consultation procedures. In this regard, the "soft" or "minor" neurological signs deserve careful review. Although the clinical significance of these signs continues to be controversial, there is increasing evidence for their utility in "signaling" a neurodevelopmental component in some child psychiatric disorders, as illustrated by the following (see also Appendix 2). When properly structured, there is a high level of test-retest reliability for soft neurological signs (6).

In well-structured cross-sectional studies, children with significant learning problems manifest certain soft signs significantly more frequently than controls (6–8).

In longitudinal studies, there is evidence for a higher number of soft signs in low birth weight children who had perinatal complications; the low birth weight children evidencing higher numbers of soft signs on follow-up at 8 years of age manifested a greater prevalence of academic and behavioral problems (9).

Boys with dysgraphesthesia and dysdiakokinesis at the age of 7 manifested a similar picture on follow-up at the age of 16 and seemed to manifest a higher prevalence of depressive symptomatology than controls (10).

Although isolated soft signs may not be of significance, the aggregate *number* of soft signs in a child can be a meaningful measure of neuroimmaturity or dysfunction (6, 8, 9).

While soft signs are often correlated with IQ (11, 12), a *combination* of both low IQ and soft signs is more highly correlated with behavioral problems.

There is increasing evidence from neuropsychological studies of higher level brain dysfunctions in psychiatric syndromes even in the presence of apparently "normal" gross neurological status (13, 14). On the other hand, definitive neurochemical and electrophysiological correlates of soft signs are not yet established. Further, clinical studies use different methods of demonstrating soft signs. However, the predominance of published findings favor some diagnostic relevance for soft or "minor" neurological signs in child and adolescent disorders. Thus, it is reasonable to hypothesize that a properly selected and structured group of these signs constituting a practical clinical instrument is in order. Most studies to date have involved a large number of items in a battery that discourages the average child psychiatrist from systematic testing. Prelimary results using a short procedure examining aspects of motor, sensory, cranial nerve, and lateralization functions appears promising. This procedure, EXAMINS (Examination for Minor Neurological Signs) is described in Appendix 2 at the end of this chapter.

However, the presence of *any one* or more of the following should lead to a traditional and comprehensive neurological examination (Appendix 1):

- Focal signs (e.g., intention tremor, weakness of a limb, weakness of one side, heightened tone of one or more of the limbs)
- Disorientation
- Evidence of a seizure disorder
- Persistent headaches
- Syncopal attacks or dizzy spells
- Recent speech impairment

- Recent impairment in memory
- Recent onset of difficulties in sphincter control
- Paralysis of a single muscle or group of muscles
- Involuntary movements
- Suspicion of a space-occupying lesion inside the calvarium
- Diplopia
- Persistent findings limited to one side or positive findings totaling more than one SD above the mean for age on administration of EXAMINS

LABORATORY INVESTIGATIONS

Laboratory procedures in child psychiatry have the advantage of being highly standardized in relation to physiological, biochemical, and structural deviations. However, they add to the expense of medical care and have to be used selectively on the basis of relevant clinical findings. They cannot substitute for a thorough and accurate clinical examination. The last decade has witnessed major growth in the available laboratory procedures in child psychiatry; the indications for and significance of current procedures are discussed below:

Complete blood count (CBC). A CBC is advisable in children who have not had one in the past 6 months. A baseline CBC is essential before starting all forms of pharmacotherapy. Clinically relevant intoxications, viral illnesses, and blood dycrasias can also be documented.

Urinary tract investigations. A basic urinalysis is indicated if not completed within the past 6 months. It is also important in every child presenting with *enuresis* to rule out urinary tract infection and diabetes mellitus. An intravenous pyelogram and voiding cystourethrogram can be helpful in identifying factors involved in daytime enuresis. Appropriate urinary tract evaluation for sexually transmitted diseases is indicated in children who have been sexually abused or have engaged in indiscriminate sexual activity.

Blood chemistry and liver profile. These tests are indicated in the work-up initiating pharmacotherapy. They are also useful in children who abuse drugs, particularly those who consume excessive amounts of alcohol, who sniff paint or glue, or who administer any drugs parenterally.

Folic acid deficiency. This test may be involved in the psychiatric disorders seen in epileptic children on anticonvulsant medications.

Radiological Studies and Neuroimaging Techniques

- When there is uncertainty on physical examination regarding presence of fecal impaction in an encopretic child, a plain x-ray of the abdomen can be helpful.
- Appropriate skull and long bone x-rays are clearly indicated in physically abused children.
- When a space-occupying lesion or other structural or vascular lesion of the brain is suspected or when increased intracranial pressure may be present, brain scan, skull x-rays, and CAT scan may be indicated. The newer neuroimaging techniques can be useful in both clinical and investigative studies. Their routine clinical use is likely to increase in the future. These techniques include the following:

Computerized Axial Tomography (CAT Scanning)

The technique of computer-assisted evaluation of x-ray data, in conjunction with the use of contrast-enhancing substances, has essentially replaced plain skull x-rays, radionuclei brain scanning, and pneumoencephalography. Brain structure is evaluated by analyzing the differential absorption of x-rays in the gray matter, white matter, and intracranial spaces containing cerebrospinal fluid. Cross-sectional images of the brain, in conjunction with the new computer programs for reconstruction of the images in any anatomic plane, allow for assessment of brain structures such as normal anatomic relationships, malformations, tumors, hemorrhages, and calcifications. This is a static study of anatomy. Information from CAT scans must be correlated with clinical and other data to assess brain function.

Positron Emission Tomography (PET Scanning)

Following the intravenous injection of biochemical tracers labeled with extremely short-lived radioactive isotopes of carbon, oxygen, and fluorine, cross-sectional quantitative autoradiographics are obtained. These images reflect regional brain metabolism or the hypermetabolic areas around actively firing seizure foci, thus extending our understanding of cerebral function. Repeated evaluations during various cognitive tasks offer dynamic information concerning brain function.

Nuclear Magnetic Resonance

NMR is the most recent advance in diagnostic brain imaging. Detailed anatomic brain images and detection of tumors, inflammation, and multiple sclerosis plaques are made possible without the use of ionizing radiation. NMR allows for a better opportunity to do detailed studies of anatomic relationships than CAT scanning.

Electroencephalogram (EEG)

The EEG has an important place in the neuropsychiatric evaluation of children. In every child manifesting unexplained temper tantrums; episodic violence; rage attacks; episodic hyperactivity; sleepy spells; vague auditory, physical, olfactory, or gustatory hallucinations; or amnesic or fugue states, an EEG with a sleep record and activating procedures of hyperventilation and photic stimulation is absolutely essential to rule out temporal-lobe-related or other seizure phenomena. The recording of cerebral electrical activity is of value in the documentation of seizures and the assessment of interictal cerebral activity. EEG is helpful in the evaluation of abnormalities of mental status due to metabolic disorders (e.g., hepatic) or infectious diseases (e.g., subacute sclerosing panencephalitis, herpes encephalitis, Creutzfeld-Jacob disease). EEG has also been used to evaluate behavioral disorders to determine whether a behavior in question may be a manifestation of a seizure disorder such as the automatisms associated with temporal lobe epilepsy. During the last several years a number of new approaches to EEG recording and advances in equipment have expanded the value of EEG in assessing disturbances in behavior. These include the following:

Prolonged EEG Recording

In order to extend the recording time, and increase the likelihood of recording abnormalities of cerebral electrical activity, prolonged EEG recording techniques have been developed. A major value is to allow for a correlation between clinical and electroencephalographic events, that is, to distinguish between episodic behavioral outbursts of a dyscontrol nature from those of temporal lobe epilepsy, and repetitive stereotyped behaviors as seen in autism from seizure phenomena. With the addition of physiologic monitors, these systems allow for recording of EKG, respirations, and eye movements, allowing for a variety of electrophysiologic and clinical correlations and for accurate sleep trend analysis (see below). Three methods are available. Although in each case the patient wears an EEG transmitter, the recording techniques differ in their method of transmitting the signal. With cable telemetry, the transmitter is connected directly to the recording device. Radioactivity telemetry permits more freedom of movement. Video monitoring via split screen may be added following the recording of the direct correlation between behavior and EEG activity. Patients undergoing these evaluations are restricted to the laboratory or hospital.

Ambulatory EEG Monitoring

Ambulatory EEG monitoring using cassette recordings allows the patient complete freedom of activity in the setting in which the EEG is recorded. The patient wears a small recording device similar to a small portable tape player. This device permits the correlation between behavior and EEG activity in the setting in which it usually occurs and observations by those who have been concerned about the behavior (e.g., by teachers in the classroom). In addition to previously mentioned values, ambulatory EEG monitoring with cassette permits evaluation of such classroom behaviors as inattentiveness by distinguishing seizure-related inattentiveness from daydreaming or deliberate avoidance behaviors. With this technique, recording of sleep studies can take place at home in a more natural setting than in a sleep laboratory.

EEG Sleep Studies

EEG recorded during prolonged periods of natural sleep allows for an evaluation of a number of sleep disorders such as sleep apnea, disorders of transitional stages (e.g., somnambulism, night terrors), and other unusual noctural events. Direct correlation with behavior can be made. A sleep trend analysis permits quantitative evaluation of sleep stages. REM sensitivity evaluations may be helpful in predicting sensitivity to tricyclic antidepressants.

Brain Electrical Activity Monitoring (BEAM)

BEAM allows for an assessment of regional brain activity. This permits a dynamic assessment during a variety of cognitive tasks such as reading and calculating. Localizing areas of dysfunction during different behavioral states may provide greater understanding of brain behavior interaction.

Neuroendocrinological Studies

The dexamethasone suppression test, while not necessary for the diagnosis of affective disorder, can be useful in the decision to use pharmacotherapy and in determining the degree of recovery and the chances for relapse (15, 16). Although clinicians utilize differing cut-off levels for cortisol, the basic test is as follows: The blood sample for cortisol level is drawn at 8:00 A.M. on day one. At 11:00 P.M. on day one the child is given either 0.5 or 1.0 mg of dexamethasone orally. Blood samples are drawn at 4:00 P.M. and 11:00 P.M. on day two for cortisol level. A cortisol level of more than 5.0 µg/dl on day two is considered positive. It is important that the laboratory establish its sensitivity for low levels of cortisol as well as the higher levels assessed. Furthermore, a positive test is not a valid indicator of neuroendocrine abnormality for up to 2 weeks after severe drug or alcohol abuse. The specificity of a positive dexamethasone suppression test for the diagnosis of depression is not as strong as it was initially thought to be.

An evaluation of thyroid function, although not routine in childhood affective disorders, may be indicated in selected patients with hyperactivity or depression based on the medical history and findings of the physical examination.

OTHER LABORATORY PROCEDURES

Neuropsychological and neurophysiological procedures such as the continuous performance test and auditory- or visual-evoked potentials are being used in research on attentional dysfunction and in learning disorders. These tools may become useful clinical procedures in the future.

- The skin conductance test does not have reliability or stability, although it is easy to perform.
- Polysomnography is a procedure that is gradually increasing in its availability and can be very useful as a diagnostic tool in sleep-related disorders.
- Chromosomal and genetic studies are indicated in the presence of a dysmorphic syndrome that deserves further delineation or when there is a strong indication of familial genetic transmission. It is advisable to call a geneticist for consultation prior to ordering these investigations.

References

1. Smith DW: Recognizable Patterns of Human Malformation, 2d ed. Philadelphia, WB Saunders Co, 1976

2. Waldrop MF, Halverson CF: Minor physical anomalies and hyperactive behavior in young children, in Exceptional Infant, Vol. 2: Studies in Abnormalities. Edited by Hellmuth J. New York, Brunner/Mazel, 1971

3. Rutter M (ed): Developmental Neuropsychiatry. New York, Guilford Press, 1983

4. Swaiman KF, Wright FS: The Practice of Pediatric Neurology, 2d ed. CV Mosby Co, St Louis, 1982

5. Menkes JH: Textbook of Child Neurology, 2d ed. Philadelphia, Lea & Febiger, 1980

6. Shaywitz SE, Shaywitz BA, McGraw K, et al: Current status of the neuromaturational examination as an index of learning disability. J Pediatr 104:819–825, 1984

7. Peters JE, Romine JS, Dykman RA: A special neurological examination of children with learning disabilities. Dev Med Child Neurol 17:63–78, 1975

8. Younes RP, Rosner B, Webb G: Neuroimmaturity of learning disabled children: a controlled study. Dev Med Child Neurol 25:574–579, 1983

9. Hertzig ME: Neurological "soft" signs in low-birth weight children. Dev Med Child Neurol 23:778–791, 1981

10. Shaffer D, O'Connor PA, Shafer SW, et al: Neurological "soft signs": their origins and significance for behavior, in Developmental Neuropsychiatry. Edited by Rutter M. New York, Guilford Press, 1983

11. Clements SD, Peters JE: Minimal brain dysfunction in the school age child. Arch Gen Psychiatry 6:185–197, 1962

12. Shaffer D: "Soft" neurological signs and later psychiatric disorder: a review. J Child Psychol Psychiatry 19:63–65, 1978

13. Golden CJ, Moses JA, Coffman JA, et al: Clinical Neuropsychology. New York, Grune & Stratton, 1983

14. Tramontana MG, Sherrets SD, Golden CJ: Brain dysfunction in youngsters with psychiatric disorders: application of the SELZ-REITAN rules for neuropsychological diagnosis. Clin Neuropsychol 2:118–124, 1980

15. Carroll BJ, Feinberg M, Greden JF, et al: A specific laboratory test for the diagnosis of melancholia: standardization, validation and clinical utility. Arch Gen Psychiatry 38:15–22, 1981

16. Leckman JF: The dexamethasone suppression test. J Am Acad Child Psychiatry 22:477–479, 1983

Appendix 1:
The Comprehensive Neurological Examination

William Singer, M.D.

Neurological examination of a child begins during the history-taking interview. At this time the behavior of the child and the interaction of parent and child can be observed. While not feeling that they are being directly examined, their fidgetiness, impulsivity, attention span, appropriateness of response to parents' comments and examiners' questions, and appropriateness of behavior in the office setting are noted. Involuntary movements such as tics and seizure activity including staring spells, eye blinking or rolling, lip smacking or other automatisms may be seen. Because these may not be noted consistently, every opportunity to observe the child should be taken.

MENTAL STATUS

Mental status testing of children should include assessments of developmental level (using standard developmental milestones and tasks) and appropriate evaluation of academic achievement (including reading, math, and spelling). Having the child copy a series of standardized geometric figures (e.g., those of Gesell) provides information concerning visual, spatial, and motor maturation and organizational skills. The ability of the child to understand and follow commands and express him- or herself verbally should also be noted. Observations should include appropriateness of speech, relevance to the setting, content, and grammar. State of alertness of the child and apparent intoxications and states of agitation or anxiety are necessary to assess the ability of the child to interact. In situations where the child is unable to cooperate with the examination, the circumstances should be noted and the examination should be repeated at a later time to provide an appropriate baseline of accomplishments.

Examination of the head includes shape, signs of trauma, defects, or bruits heard with the stethoscope over the eyes. Scaphocephalic appearance of the head is commonly seen in children who are premature neonates. A flattened occiput over which the hair is sparse or absent may indicate a child who has spent a great deal of time lying on his or her back with limited amounts of stimulation. Irregularities of head shape relevant to premature suture closure may also be seen. Single suture synostosis is of cosmetic significance only. Signs of trauma including battle sign and raccoon sign are significant in assessing the mental status of the child as well as their appropriateness of interaction.

CRANIAL NERVE EXAMINATION

Cranial Nerve I (olfactory nerve). Each nostril is tested separately using substances such as peppermint or vanilla. Anosmia may be due to intercurrent upper respiratory tract infection or sinusitis but may also be seen following head trauma or in conjunction with subfrontal tumors compressing the olfactory nerves.

Cranial Nerve II (optic nerve). Visual acuity is assessed using standard Snellen charts. Visual fields are tested by confrontation. Funduscopic examination is done to assess presence of papilledema (increased intercranial pressure), optic atrophy (usually associated with a history of change in visual acuity), and optic hypoplasia. Retinas may reveal healed choreo-retinitis, suggesting intrauternine infection or active retinitis associated with current infection. An absence of pigment is associated with albinism. In patients presenting with headaches or changes in behavior, a funduscopic examination is extremely important.

Cranial Nerves III, IV, and VI. These nerves innervate the extraocular muscles. Common eye deviations include phorias (eyes are straight during fixation but deviate when one eye is covered) and tropias (deviations are not affected by fixation). Such abnormalities are commonly seen in infants and children. They are of increasing importance when they develop as a new sign in a previously asymptomatic child. Failure of the eyes to deviate laterally (cranial nerve VI weakness) may be a nonlocalizing sign of increased intracranial pressure. Head tilt may develop in an effort to restore visual fusion when a deficit in extraoccular movement develops. It may also be seen in cerebellar hemisphere tumors without abnormalities of extraocular movements. Extraocular muscle movement abnormalities may be seen in congenital muscle weakness, severe visual impairment, increased intracranial pressure, pontine tumors, myasthenia gravis, or ophthalmoplegic migraine. Lesions of cranial nerve III may produce an ipsilateral ptosis as well as eye deviation. Pupils are tested with direct and consensual light.

Cranial Nerve V (trigeminal nerve). The sensory divisions innervate the face, anterior one-half of the scalp, and the cornea. Motor divisions innervate muscles of mastication. Motor dysfunction results in deviation of the jaw to one side of the lesion on opening.

Cranial Nerve VII (facial nerve). The motor division innervates facial muscles while sensory fibers supply taste fibers to the anterior two-thirds of the tongue. Lesions of the facial nucleus or peripheral nerve result in weakness of all facial movement on the side of the lesion. Central facial weakness results in the weakness of the facial muscles with preservation of forehead wrinkling. Taste-testing is possible with a variety of substances.

Cranial Nerve VIII (auditory nerve). This nerve consists

of auditory and vestibular divisions. Gross assessment of auditory function is made by observing the appropriateness of response to directions and questions, paying close attention to the child's speech. A lack of speech sounds, and poorly articulated speech in younger children suggests a hearing impairment. Full audiometric testing should be done. Children with behavioral disturbances and delayed language development must have an assessment of hearing function. Dysfunction of the vestibular nerve is suggested by a history of vertigo and gait disturbance. It may be seen in conjunction with acquired developmental delay, new onset of behavioral disturbance, and clumsiness of motor function following head trauma or central nervous system infection.

Cranial Nerves IX and X (glossopharyngeal and vagus nerves). These nerves innervate the palate, pharynx, and larynx. Lesions will result in ipsilateral paralysis of the pharyngeal muscles with an inability of the soft palate to elevate on gag. Bilateral lesions cause nasality of speech and fluids to regurgitate into the nasal pharynx during attempts to swallow.

Cranial Nerve XI (spinal accessory nerve). This nerve innervates the sternocleidomastoid and trapezius muscles. Dysfunction of the sternocleidomastoid muscles is indicated by an inability to turn the head to the opposite side. Dysfunction of the trapezius muscle results in a shoulder droop and inability to shrug ipsilaterally.

Cranial Nerve XII (hypoglossal nerve). This nerves innervates the tongue. Unilateral lesions result in a deviation of the protruded tongue to the involved side. Lesions result in atrophy and fasciculation on the ipsilateral side. Bilateral lesions result in a relatively immobile tongue, severe dysarthria, and inability to protrude the tongue beyond the teeth.

MOTOR SYSTEM

Muscle strength in any extremity is assessed by testing individual or groups of muscles against resistance. Strength is graded using the guidelines of the Medical Research Council (Memorandum #7): 0 = no muscle control; 1 = trace muscle contraction; 2 = active movement at joint, effects of gravity removed; 3 = active movement of joint, against gravity; 4 = active movement of joint, against resistance; 5 = normal (4, 5). In young or cooperative children, a functional assessment of muscle strength testing large muscle groups rather than individual muscle testing may be obtained during game playing or motor tasks such as walking, stair climbing, running, or supporting the body in a wheelbarrow position. Symmetry and contour of the muscle mass is assessed by inspection. Unilateral muscle wasting and underdevelopment of an extremity is often seen in early cerebral lesions and may be the only indication of a mild hemiparesis. Atrophy with fasciculations is seen in anterior horn disease. Calf hypertrophy is seen in Duchenne's muscular dystrophy.

Tone is the resistance of muscles to passive movement while at rest. Hypotonia (decreased tone) is seen in myopathies, anterior horn cell disorders, peripheral neuropathies, and cerebellar disorders. Hypertonia (increased tone) is characteristic of central nervous system disorders (brain or spinal cord) affecting the cortical spinal tracts.

Rigidity is characteristic of extrapyramidal disorders whether medication-induced or due to primary central nervous system dysfunction. The tone may be continuously increased (lead pipe rigidity) or interrupted by ratchet-like movements (cog wheel rigidity).

Deep tendon reflexes are routinely tested in the biceps, triceps, brachioradialis, patella, and Achilles tendons. Grading is as follows: 0 = areflexia; 1 = hyporeflexia; 2 = normal; 3 = hyperreflexia; 4 = clonus. Generalized hyperreflexia may be seen in anxious children as well as in central nervous system disorders affecting the muscle and peripheral nerve.

Plantar response is elicited by distally moving noxious stimulus along the lateral margin of the foot. After the neonatal period, the normal response of the great toe is plantar flexion. Extension of the great toe with fanning of the other toes (Babinski sign) is indicative of cortical spinal tract dysfunction.

Cerebellar Examination. Regulation and coordination are felt to be functions of the cerebellum. Lesions of the cerebeller vermis result in truncal ataxia with disturbance of gait and sitting balance. Lesions of the cerebellar hemisphere are characterized by limb ataxia accompanied by tremor during active movement with terminal accentuation and loss of rhythmicity of repetitive movements. Speech is poorly articulated and explosive, often accompanied by stuttering. Cerebellar testing consists of finger-to-nose and heel-to-shin testing, repetitive heel shin tapping, rapid finger apposition, alternating pronation of hands and forearms, as well as observation of gait. Romberg maneuver is usually negative.

Disorders of movement. Chorea (brief, very rapid movements of proximal and distal muscle groups). Lesion is in the corpus striatum (caudate nucleus). Juvenile Huntington's disease may present with chorea before behavioral changes occur. Sydenham's chorea may cause behavioral adjustment difficulties if its course is prolonged.

Tremor. Rhythmic movements usually involving distal muscles of the extremities. Tremors of cerebellar origin are usually present during volitional movements exacerbated at the terminus of the movement. Extrapyramidal tremors are characterized by pill-rolling movement of the hands at rest, subsiding during volitional movements. Tremors of Wilson's disease (associated with hepatic dysfunction) involve muscles of shoulder girdle and proximal upper extremities (wing-beating tremor). Central nervous system stimulants (e.g., cocaine and amphetamines) result in a rapid, fine, limb tremor.

Athetosis. Slow writhing movements most prominent in distal muscle groups but also involving promixal portions of the extremities as well as head and neck. Lesions of the globus pallidus are responsible for athetosis.

Hemiballism. Flailing, often with flinging movements of the extremities of one side. Lesions of the subthalamic nucleus of Luey are responsible.

Torsional Dystonia. Slow rotatory repetitive movements involving the head, neck, and trunk. Lesions of the putamen are implicated.

Spastic Torticollis. Rotatory movements limited to head and neck.

Myoclonus. Sudden jerking movements of individual muscle groups.

Gait and Station. The child is observed moving about in the examining room. Base should be narrow and gait should be steady heel-toe progression. Disturbances may be due to lesions of central or peripheral nervous systems. Running should be observed since it serves to exaggerate abnormalities or gait.

- *Cerebellar gait*: A wide ataxic gait. As the base is narrowed (e.g., tandem walking) the gait becomes more disordered. This type of gait does not deteriorate with eye closure (negative Romberg sign).
- *Steppage gait*: Suggests a peripheral nerve abnormality. Such disorders result in foot drop either unilaterally or bilaterally. As joint sensation is compromised, the loss of visual cues to foot position during eye closure results in deterioration of gait (Romberg sign is positive).
- *Spastic gait*: Characteristically increased adduction of the hips results in a stiff-legged circumducting gait with limited flexion at the hip and knee and toe walking. This may be unilateral or bilateral.
- *Waddling gait*: Suggests proximal muscle weakness involving pelvic girdle and trunk muscles, as is seen in the muscular dystrophies and anterior horn cell diseases.

Sensory Systems

The sensory examination is the most difficult part of the neurological examination. The success of sensory testing varies with the cooperation of the subject and the age (maturity) of the child. Position and vibration sense should be tested in all extremities. Abnormalities may be seen in lesions affecting posterior columns of the spinal cord or peripheral nerves. Touch, single and double simultaneous stimulation, and pinprick are included in the examination. Sensory abnormalities may reflect segmental deficits or those of peripheral or cutaneous nerve origin.

Corticosensory testing evaluates sensory pathways from the peripheral sensory systems to the parietal lobe. The following functions are assessed.

- Graphesthesia—identification of numbers written on the skin of the palm, forearm, and dorsum of the foot. By 8 years of age the child should be able to recognize all numbers to 9. Loss = dysgraphesthesia.
- Stereognosis—identification of familiar objects (e.g., keys and coins) by touch using size, form, and texture. Loss = astereognosis = parietal lobe dysfunction.
- Tapagnosis—ability to localize tactile stimuli. Loss = atapagnosis = cortical lesion.
- Double simultaneous stimulation—perception of being touched on two parts of the body simultaneously. Failure to perceive = lesion of parietal lobe.
- Two-point discrimination—test of minimal distance between two simultaneously applied cutaneous stimuli. Asymmetry is seen in unilateral parietal lobe dysfunction.

Appendix 2:
Examination for Minor Neurological Signs (EXAMINS)

P. S. B. Sarma, M.B., B.S.

In this procedure, 18 items are scored on a dichotomous basis and the neurological impairment index is calculated by adding the number of positive items in the child. The test manifests satisfactory test–retest reliability (mean κ score of 0.76), neuromaturational sensitivity (as manifested by a correlation of -0.5 or above in more than one study between the impairment index and age), and discriminant ability in identifying academically impaired boys (with low false positives) in the 7- to 10-year age range.* The number of positive items in each age group in a sample of 70 well-functioning children aged 6 to 10 years is listed in Table 1. Any child of either sex who scores 1 SD above the mean for that age is likely to have significant neurocognitive or neurobehavioral impairment. This test manifests potential utility as a screening instrument to select children for more complex and time-consuming neuropsychological and neurological investigations.

Any time a child fails a particular test of this group, the test is repeated. Only if the test is failed a second time is it marked as fail or impaired. No feedback is given to the child until the test is completed.

---

*Data from papers presented at the annual meetings of the American Academy of Child Psychiatry in 1983 and 1984. These data reflect the initial descriptions of one systematic approach to the evaluation of soft signs. They are presented to guide the beginning clinician and will require replication and time before gaining broad clinical usage.

1. Arm Dominance. The examiner asks the child to demonstrate throwing an imaginary baseball. Then the examiner asks the child to write his or her name. If there is any uncertainty, the child is asked to demonstrate these activities with each arm so the examiner can determine which side is better in each task.
Pass: If there is a clear dominance of the same arm for both of these activities. The side of arm dominance is recorded.

2. Leg Preference. The examiner asks the child to demonstrate kicking a ball and hopping on one foot. If there is any doubt, the child is asked to demonstrate three or four times. The choice of the same leg for kicking and for hopping is looked for.
Pass: If there is a clear preference of the leg on the same side as the arm or if the leg preference is unclear.

3. Eye Dominance. The examiner sits on a chair facing the child and demonstrates holding one sheet of paper in each hand (held by the outer edge of the sheet) in front of his or her face and then focusing on the child's nose while moving the two sheets of paper slowly toward the midline until the view is blocked out. Then the child is asked to repeat this process a few times. The examiner makes sure that the child is not resting an arm or elbow on an arm rest or table while performing this task. The examiner observes if one eye of the child is consistently blocked by the paper first and the other eye of the child is visible to the examiner almost until the end. The eye that is covered last in a consistent manner (four

Table 1. Results of Examination for Minor Neurological Signs in 70 Well-Functioning Children

Age	N	Mean ± SD No. of Positive Items
6	13	6.3 ± 1.18
7	12	4.17 ± 1.69
8	21	3.85 ± 1.35
9	17	2.88 ± 1.93
10	7	1.71 ± 1.49

out of six times) is considered the dominant eye.
Pass: If the dominant eye is on the same side as the dominant hand or if there is no clearcut dominance of one eye over the other.

4. Digit Span. The child is instructed that the examiner will say some numbers and the child is to repeat them in the same order after the examiner finishes. Then an example is given (1,2,3). Then the examiner starts with a three-number series and proceeds as follows with three tests at each level to six numbers. About ½-second intervals are given between numbers.

$$
\begin{array}{c}
6,1,8 \\
3,2,5 \\
\hline
8,3,5,1 \\
7,4,9,3 \\
5,3,1,8 \\
\hline
1,4,8,6,3 \\
7,9,3,1,5 \\
3,9,5,1,6 \\
\hline
5,7,9,6,4,2 \\
1,5,8,4,3,9 \\
\hline
\end{array}
$$

Pass: (a) If the child recalls all the five-digit series or (b) if the child makes one mistake in the five-digit series but is able to recall at least one of the six-digit series.

5. Speech. The child is engaged in sufficient informal conversation to permit the assessment of clarity and intelligibility. Then the child is asked to repeat: "Washington," "Kentucky," "Oklahoma," "Wisconsin," "Massachusetts," "Pennsylvania," "Virginia."
Pass: If the child repeats all but one of the statements clearly, the way it was said.

6. Visual Tracking. The child is asked to follow the top of a pen or pencil (held about 12 inches from his or her face) with the eyes without turning the head. The pencil is moved such that lateral gaze on each side to a 60-degree angle is tested. Irregular ocular pursuit, jerky movements while crossing the midline, and any persistent overshooting or undershooting is looked for.
Pass: If the ocular pursuit is smooth without persistent overshooting or undershooting.

7. Eye Symmetry. Symmetry of the eyes during visual tracking and during alternate focusing on a distant object and on a pencil held about 3 inches in front of the forehead is looked for.
Pass: If there is no symmetry on lateral gaze or during convergence.

8. Nystagmus. During the above test nystagmus or consistent nystagmoid movements of 4 beats or more during lateral gaze are looked for.
Pass: If there are no consistent nystagmoid jerks of 4 beats or more during lateral gaze.

9. Right–Left Identification on Self. The child is asked to raise the left hand, to touch the right ear, left shoulder, and right knee.
Pass: If the child is correct four of the four times.

10. Right-Left Identification on Examiner. The examiner faces the child, holds his or her own (examiner's) hands out in front and asks the child "Which is my right hand?" "Which is my left hand?" Then the examiner crosses his or her forearms in front and again asks the above questions.
Pass: If the child is correct four of the four times.

11. Bilateral Hand Stimulation. This test is generally passed by all children older than age 5, and it serves as a screening test to determine if the child will be able to cooperate reliably in the following four sensory tests. If the child is unable to pass this test, it is very unlikely that the child's responses to the following four tests will be reliable.

The child is asked to place his or her hands on the table with palms down. The child is told that he or she will be touched on one hand at a time or on both hands at the same time (with demonstration of each category of touch). The child is told to keep eyes closed and to state "one" or "both" when the touch is felt. Both hands are touched four times simultaneously with some episodes of single touch interposed.

Pass: If the child identifies all the episodes of touch correctly.

12. *Finger Localization.* The child is asked to place hands on the table with palms down and fingers spread. The child is told that one of his or her fingers will be touched lightly and this is demonstrated with a light stroke (lasting about ½ second) on the dorsum of the proximal phalanx of one of the fingers. Then the child is asked to close the eyes. One of the middle fingers is touched. The child is then asked to open the eyes and point to the finger that was touched. (The thumb and little finger are not touched because they are fairly easy to identify.) After the six trials of single finger touch are completed, the child is told that now two fingers will be touched simultaneously and they may be right next to each other or separated by a finger in between. Again, three trials on each hand involving the different combinations of the three fingers are performed.

Pass: If the child makes no more than one mistake in the whole test involving 12 trials.

13. *Face–Hand Test.* The child is asked to place hands on the table palms down. The child is then told that he or she may be touched on the hand (a light stroke lasting about ½ second on the dorsum of the hand) or on the cheek or both hand and cheek. The child is then told to close the eyes and to state where he or she is touched when the touch is felt. The cheek and hand on each side are touched simultaneously four times with either hand only or cheek only touch interposed.

Pass: If child identifies the simultaneous touches of hand and cheek with no more than one mistake of omission (e.g., fails to identify when both hand and cheek are touched) and no more than one mistake of commission (e.g., states "hand and cheek" when only hand or cheek is touched).

14. Graphesthesia. First the examiner writes the following numbers on the table with the blunt end of the pen so that the child is familiar with the way 2, 3, 4, 6, 7, and 8 are written by the examiner. Then the child is asked to place hands on the table with palms up, to keep the eyes closed, and to guess what numbers are being written in different order alternately in each hand.
Pass: If the child makes no more than one mistake in the whole test involving 12 trials.

15. Stereognosis. The child is first made familiar with the visual identification of the three items involved: button, quarter, and penny. Then the child is told to keep eyes closed and to figure out which one of the three objects is placed in his or her hand. The child is asked to place hands on the table palms up and to close the eyes. Then one item at a time is placed in the child's palm and the child is encouraged to feel the size and shape of the object without transferring the object to the other hand and guess what the item is. The maximum time allowed for each trial is 10 seconds. The objects are placed alternately in each hand in a different order so that each object is placed at least twice in each hand.
Pass: If the child makes no more than one mistake in the whole test involving 12 trials (two trials for each object in each hand).

16. Finger-to-Nose Test. The examiner first demonstrates to the child how to touch the tip of one's nose with the tip of an index finger after fully extending the arm initially. The child is then asked to do the same with each hand twice. When the child is able to do this, the child is asked to do so five times with each hand, with eyes closed.
Pass: If the child is able to perform this test without significant tremors or past pointing. Failure in this test usually indicates

the need for a traditional neurological evaluation.

17. *Diadokokinesis*. The process of tapping the table with the palm and the dorsum of the hand alternately is demonstrated to the child and the child is encouraged to practice it for about 10 seconds with each hand. Then the child is asked to do it with the right hand as rapidly as possible. The examiner counts the number of times the child taps the table with the palm in 10 seconds. The procedure is then repeated with the left hand.
Pass: If the child taps the table with each palm at least 12 times in 10 seconds.

18. *Synkinesias*. The child stands facing the examiner. With an arm flexed at the elbow to 90 degrees, the child is asked to pretend twisting an imaginery doorknob back and forth. This is demonstrated to the child by the examiner. The examiner observes for movement of the child's fingers or hand on the opposite side. The procedure is repeated with the other hand.

19. *Passive Head Turning*. The child is helped to stand comfortably with feet slightly apart and with the arms held out in front at the shoulder level with the fingers spread. Then the child is told that the examiner will stand behind the child and turn the child's head from side to side. The child is instructed to leave his or her head loose so that the examiner can turn it but not to let the arms or body turn. The head is turned to each side from the midline from side to side. If the child appears to be voluntarily moving the head, the child is instructed not to assist the examiner but to leave the head loose. The freedom to move the head in a 160-degree range is assessed. The examiner also observes the hands to see if either hand crosses the midline when the head is turned.
Pass: If both the following criteria are met: (a) there is no significant resistance to passive turning of the head and (b) neither hand crosses the midline while the head is being turned.

Chapter 4

Psychological Testing

Sid Mondell, Ph.D.

Terrell Clark, Ph.D.

Psychological testing is an important component of the child's diagnostic evaluation and a complement to other sources of data. Testing is also used in school or vocational assessments, pretreatment baseline evaluations, and for a variety of research purposes. There are several forms of psychological testing, including:

- Cognitive (IQ) tests,
- Educational (achievement) tests,
- Tests of visual motor skills,
- Children's drawing tests,
- Projective personality tests, and
- Neuropsychological tests (1–4).

Psychological tests distinguish themselves from other forms of interview data through their attention to standardized administration, use of reference or norm groups, and the presence of carefully researched studies of their reliability and validity.

The skills and knowledge necessary for the administration

and interpretation of these tests require extensive training and clinical experience. "Psychologists" or "professional psychologists" refer to a doctoral level (Ph.D., Ed.D., or Psy.D.) professional who has received a degree from a regionally accredited graduate school in the fields of clinical, counseling, educational, or school psychology. Although the term "psychologist" may be used loosely, the careful clinician is urged to collaborate with professionals with the highest levels of training, education, and experience.

Psychological testing has its historical roots in World War I when research studies on the nature of intelligence led to the development of test instruments. The U.S. "Army Alpha" test was such a prototype and was used to sort out quickly the suitability of men being conscripted into the military services. Since that time, the concept of standardized tests to sort, type, or describe people relative to some reference group has flourished. Psychological research led to the evolution of the tests used today and continues to develop, paving the way for new formats and revisions of existing tests that will be used tomorrow. As people, times, and reference groups change, so must these instruments.

INDICATIONS FOR USE OF PSYCHOLOGICAL TESTING

In general, the indications for or advantages of using psychological testing as part of the diagnostic evaluation of children include the following:

- In particularly complex and complicated diagnostic evaluations, psychological testing provides data of a qualitatively different nature from interviews and history. The additional data, with reference to norm groups, standardization, and objective or quantitative scoring, may shed new light and contribute valuable pieces to the diagnostic puzzle. In some cases testing may reaffirm impressions gleaned from other sources of information; in other instances it may raise new questions, concerns, a child's hidden strengths, or sus-

pected but unconfirmed vulnerabilities that were not obtained in prior evaluation.
- Some diagnostic information (e.g., IQ, cognitive functioning, educational achievement, the presence of learning disability) is definitively assessed *only* by psychological testing. Although mental status evaluation or interview may suggest estimates, actual quantitative scores may be obtained only through competently administered testing.
- Psychological testing may be required or mandated by law. P.L. 94-142, or its state equivalent, which mandates individual educational planning for the handicapped student, requires psychological testing specifically to assess cognitive, educational, and psychological functioning.
- In forensic evaluations, courts and lawyers often favor testing and quantitative scores. Testing is often perceived by courts as more "objective" due to a standardization of administration, scoring, and interpretations.
- Testing is often helpful in persuading parents to accept treatment recommendations or diagnostic impressions of their child. The perception of objectivity and standardization can help in such situations.
- Test data are often useful in establishing a quantitative or "objective" baseline for a child before some changes (educational, social, or therapeutic) are introduced.

Psychological testing is generally perceived by children and adolescents as a pleasant, helpful, or even growth-enhancing experience. Most children enjoy the testing experience and "feel good" or even relieved at its completion. At times, symptom improvement results following the testing, a so-called testing cure. Improvement may result from placing appropriate attention and concern on a previously neglected problem. In other cases, psychological testing and follow-up feedback to the parents and the child leaves an individual or family system ripe for therapeutic interventions by again drawing appropriate attention and concern to problems requiring further work, recognition, or elucidation.

LIMITATIONS OF TESTING

Included among the limitations of psychological testing are the following:

- Not all testing may be given to all children. Tests vary as to specific age ranges and appropriate references or standardization in regard to age or other relevant characteristics.
- Tests generally have lower reliability and thus are less valid with preschool children (below age 6). One must qualify test results with these children and take into account various factors that may have lowered or altered a given "performance" relative to the child's true competence or "inherent nature."
- Testing in general is highly language dependent. Thus its usefulness is more limited with children who have major verbal handicaps, who are preverbal, or who speak a primary language different from the psychological tester. Some specific tests are less language dependent (e.g., Peabody Picture Vocabulary Test-Revised). Interpretation must be made cautiously in all cases of language impairment or concern.
- Testing can be frightening and perceived as overly intrusive or humiliating by a minority of children and, especially, their parents. Timing administration and recommendations become important in such instances.
- Testing can be "forced" or administered without the active cooperation and participation of the child.
- If a child becomes mute, obstinate, or otherwise uncooperative, valid test results cannot be obtained. Children who are in altered states of consciousness, who are heavily sedated or medicated, or who are in physical restraints cannot be tested.
- Children should not be "overtested." Retesting within one year's time is rarely optimal and may prove invalid because of practice effects. Annual testing is a similar misuse of psychological testing. Prior consultation before referral with

a professional psychologist is recommended where the advisability of testing, given a previous record of testing for the child, is questioned.
- Psychological testing, although often covered by mental health insurance policies, is an expensive procedure. For every hour of administration with the child present, a psychologist may spend another 1 to 3 hours scoring, interpreting, and writing up results. This time investment results in relatively high costs that must be individually weighed against the need and the patient's family's ability to afford the service.

COGNITIVE ASSESSMENT

The appraisal of children's intellectual functioning plays an important role in clinical child psychology. What is actually measured through intelligence testing and what comprises "intelligence" is a source of both academic and political controversy. There is a strong positive correlation between measured IQ and achievement in school. The development and exercise of cognitive abilities and learning go hand-in-hand for most children. In conducting intelligence testing, a well-trained, qualified clinical psychologist will observe the child's manner, style, behaviors, responses, and appearance. How the child executes items on the test instruments and how the child relates to the examiner are diagnostically important, and bear on the evaluation as much as how well the child scores on the tests administered.

There are a number of individually administered tests of intellectual functioning used in clinical practice. The most popular and widely used of these are the Wechsler scales, which have three versions. The Wechsler Preschool and Primary Scale of Intelligence (WPPSI) is appropriate for use with young children ages 4 to 6. The Wechsler Intelligence Scale for Children-Revised (WISC-R) is designed for youngsters ages 6 to 16. For those ages 16 and over, the Wechsler Adult Intelligence Scale-Revised (WAIS-R) is used.

The Wechsler scales are among the best of intelligence tests available for clinical use. Their reliability and validity have proven to be stable over time in comparison with other respected tests of intellectual functioning and academic achievement. The Wechsler scales are composed of a number of subtests, some of which emphasize knowledge of vocabulary, auditory comprehension, and verbal reasoning. Others rely more heavily on visually presented information and manipulation of pictures, puzzles, and objects in largely nonverbal reasoning, perceptual, organizational, and problem-solving tasks. Scores yielded on the Wechsler scales include a Verbal Intelligence Quotient, Performance Intelligence Quotient, and Full Scale Intelligence Quotient, as well as incrementally comparable scaled scores for each of the individual subtests. The following summaries provide a description of the subtests of the WISC-R:

Verbal Scale Subtests

Information: Assesses familiarity with basic facts in topics such as history, geography, and science.
Similarities: Assesses logic, verbal reasoning, and ability to explain associations and relationships.
Arithmetic: Requires solution of so-called word problems through mental computation without paper and pencil.
Vocabulary: Requires explanation or formulation of definitions of the meaning of words.
Comprehension: Assesses responses to questions regarding exercise of common sense, social judgment, and practical knowledge.
Digit Span: An alternate or optional subtest in which repetition of random series of numbers is required.

Performance Scale Subtests

Picture Completion: Involves ability to differentiate essential from nonessential details and visual memory as well as recognition of pictures of common objects and animals.
Picture Arrangement: Involves sequencing of pictures into logical order and involves ability to note cause–effect

relationships and to interpret social situations.

Block Design: Perceptual–organizational skills, reasoning, and problem-solving abilities are required to reproduce geometric patterns using colored cubes.

Object Assembly: Involves perception of part–whole relationships; manipulation of puzzle pieces; and problem-solving, organizational, and visual–spatial skills.

Coding: Speed and accuracy of performance are measured in this paper-and-pencil task involving associational learning and manipulation of arbitrary visual symbols.

Mazes: An alternate or optional subtest involving visual–motor planning and integration skills.

The WPPSI and WAIS-R are composed of similar types of tasks and subtests. The titles of the subtests on these scales differ slightly. Naturally, the levels of item difficulty are designed to challenge individuals in their respective age groups. On all versions of the Wechsler scales, the average scaled score is 10. Scaled scores above 7 and below 13 comprise the average range. Very low values would be in the range of 1 to 3 and very high values would be those above 16.

Two relatively new tests of cognitive development and intellectual functioning are gaining in popularity among psychologists for use with very young children. These are the McCarthy Scales of Children's Abilities and the Kaufman-Assessment Battery for Children. The Merrill-Palmer Scale of Mental Tests and the newer Extended Merrill-Palmer Scale are also widely used in the assessment of preschool-aged children.

To augment diagnostic information gained from administration of the more comprehensive tests of intelligence, such as the Wechsler scales or the Stanford-Binet Intelligence Scale, psychologists might choose also to examine vocabulary development, sophistication of human figure drawings, or responses on brief screening measures. Tests utilized for these purposes might include the Peabody Picture Vocabulary Test-Revised, Goodenough-Harris Drawing Test, Developmental Test of Visual-Motor Integration (VMI), Slosson Intelligence Test, and Ammons Quick Test.

Children who display extraordinary physical or mental disabilities (e.g., blindness or visual impairment, deafness or hearing impairment, cerebral palsy, severe mental retardation, infantile autism, extreme language and communication disorders) often demand extraordinary skills on the part of the psychologist conducting the evaluation. Some of the more specialized tests that might be utilized include the Leiter International Performance Scale, Columbia Mental Maturity Scale, Progressive Matrices, Pictorial Test of Intelligence, Haptic Intelligence Test for Adult Blind, and Hiskey-Nebraska Test of Learning Aptitude. Not all psychologists are experienced in administering and interpreting results from these tests, nor in evaluation of youngsters with such handicaps.

What types of diagnostic information can be obtained from tests of cognitive development and intellectual functioning? One type of score is an intelligence quotient (IQ). Normative data from most tests have been statistically manipulated such that the "average" IQ is 100. Scores within one standard deviation of the mean are considered to fall within the average range. Scores which differ from the mean by more than one standard deviation (in either direction) are considered to be significant and thereby indicative of relative strengths and/or weaknesses.

There are various classifications of intelligence offered by authors of these intelligence tests. Generally, the levels of classification parallel those outlined in Table 1.

Another type of score that may be obtained is a mental age

Table 1. Classifications of Intelligence as Measured by IQ Tests

Measured IQ	Classification	Incidence
≥130	Very superior	Top 2% of population
120–129	Superior	
110–119	Bright or high average	
90–109	Average	Middle 50% of population
80–89	Dull or low average	
70–79	Borderline	
<70	Mentally defective	Bottom 2% of population
50–69	Mild retardation	
25–49	Moderate retardation	
<20–24	Severe retardation	

(MA) or age equivalency (AE) score. Understanding the concept of MA is intricate. The relationship between MA and chronological age is not a static one. That a 3-year-old earns an MA of 4 years may be indicative of superior level intellectual potential, whereas an 11-year-old passing tests at the 12-year-age equivalency level may simply be demonstrating average level functioning. Also, a mentally retarded individual 15 years of age who earns an MA of 8 years is not likely to resemble a typical third grader in learning style, intellectual curiosity, or repertoire of functional and adaptive skills. There is usefulness to the notion of age equivalency scores, but their meaning requires interpretation and explanation by an experienced clinician.

Analyses of results from various tests administered and of responses to items within various segments of given tests yield valuable information regarding cognitive ability, learning style, and relative talents and deficits. The ability to interpret test protocols and profiles is the key area of expertise for skilled psychologists. One needs to understand more than a global estimate of cognitive ability (the IQ) when psychological testing is requested for a child. The influence of factors such as ethnic and family background, educational experiences, emotional adjustment, physical disabilities, organic impairments, specific learning disorders, and environment must be considered. The contribution of such factors is often reflected in the content of children's responses and revealed in analysis of the results of testing.

Although comprehensive assessment of cognitive skills is necessary in many clinical situations, an office screening of these functions can be a useful diagnostic tool. Such a screening device should never substitute for a full scale study but can be taught to the beginning child psychiatrist by an experienced clinical psychologist. One new approach to this task is described in Appendix 1 at the end of this chapter.

ACADEMIC SKILLS

All children should have entered school by the age of 6. Although many begin formal educational experiences at age 3 or 4, most participate in some kind of kindergarten experience, either public or private. A simple way to determine what grade a child "should" be in is to subtract 5 from the child's chronological age. Thereby, 6-year-olds are generally first graders, 8-year-olds are third graders, and so on.

School is the consuming arena in which children between the ages of 5 or 6 and 16 to 18 must grow, prove themselves, flourish, and succeed. Failures experienced in school are likely to be dramatically expressed in other spheres of the child's life. Likewise, trauma, disappointment, illness, upset, anger, anxiousness, and defeat in any aspect of a child's existence usually spills over into the school setting and affects academic, social, and interpersonal performance there. Understanding the school experience of children is therefore crucial to effective diagnosis and treatment of this age group.

At no age is school seen as merely a playground. Both from the children's and the teachers' points of view, the responsibility of schooling is far more serious than that. There are rules to be obeyed and there are lessons to be learned. Beginning with shapes, colors, letters, numbers, community helpers, animal products, and parts of the body, the content of curricula quickly escalates to the complexities of grammar, set theory, main ideas, supporting details, world geography, dates in history, chemical structures, and transportation and communication systems. The demands on 7-year-olds in the classroom would astound most adults. Even so, the majority of children capably meet these demands and perform at least adequately in the school setting.

Although one encounters variations among local school districts, the following represents a fairly typical curricular progression through the elementary grades:

Kindergarten

- Recognizing, naming, and forming letters
- Spelling and printing first and last name
- Counting at least to 20
- Recognizing, naming, and forming shapes

- Identifying (by name and function) instruments such as clock, calendar, thermometer, and ruler

First Grade

- Reading
- Beginning phonics (short vowels, long vowels, single consonants)
- Basal texts
  - Preprimer (50–75 words)
  - Primer (100–175 words)
  - First-grade level reader (250–350 words)

- Comprehension skills
  - Story titles
  - Locating specific facts or information

- Spelling and writing
  - Common spelling rules or conventions
  - Mastery of approximately 100 words
  - Recognizing and printing letters

- Math
  - Counting at least to 50
  - Simple addition and subtraction
  - Simple fractions (½, ⅓, ¼)
  - Telling time by the hour
  - Naming values of coins

Second Grade

- Reading
  - 2^1 and 2^2 level readers (950–1700 words)

- Phonics, including consonant blends and digraphs (e.g., ch, st, ck), vowel digraphs (e.g., ai, ea, oa), and r-controlled vowels (e.g., ar, ir).
- Comprehension skills
  - Main idea

- Sequence of events
  - Author's intent

- Spelling and writing
  - Mastery of approximately 300 words
  - Correct formation and spacing of all uppercase and lowercase letters

- Math
  - Counting by 2s and 10s
  - Reading 2-digit numerals
  - Column 2-digit numerals
  - Column addition and subtraction
  - Place value
  - Telling time by hour, half-hour, and quarter-hour
  - Fractions ($2/3$, $5/8$)
  - Measuring by the inch and half-inch and/or by centimeters

Third Grade

- Reading
  - 3^1 and 3^2 level readers (1900–3300 words)

- Mastery of phonics
- Structural analysis (prefixes, suffixes, roots)
- Decoding skills
- Comprehension skills
  - Describing skills
  - Anticipating conclusions
  - Comparing authors' styles

- Spelling and handwriting
  - Cursive writing introduced
  - Short compositions and formal letters of correspondence
  - Use of dictionary and alphabetization
  - Spelling rules: formation of plurals, common phonograms, affixes (change of verb tense, adding "ly")

- Math
  - Counting by 3s and 5s
  - Identifying 3-digit and 4-digit numerals (100s and 1000s)
  - Adding and subtracting with regrouping (carrying and borrowing)
  - Simple multiplication
  - Finding lowest common denominator among fractions
  - Adding sums of money and making change

Fourth Grade

- Reading
  - Fourth-grade level reader (2800–3500 words)
  - Emphasis shifts from oral to silent reading
  - Having "learned to read," priority becomes "reading to learn"
  - Comprehension and content become most important

- Spelling and writing
  - Exclusive use of cursive style handwriting
  - Approximately 2000 spelling words mastered
  - Considerable written production expected (compositions, reports, term projects)

- Math
  - Roman numerals
  - Times tables committed to memory
  - Division introduced

Fifth Grade

- Reading
  - Fifth-grade level reader (4500–6000 words)
  - Study skills emphasized (outlining, summarizing, note taking)
  - Rate or speed of silent reading increases

- Spelling and writing
  - Proofreading and self-correction of spelling and punctuation
  - Continued emphasis on reports, compositions, projects, essays
  - Volume of written output increases considerably

- Math
  - Division with remainders
  - Computations with fractions
  - Geometric principles (diameter, area, polygons)
  - Use of instruments (metric ruler, compass, barometer)
  - Units of measure (equivalents and conversion)

Sixth Grade

- Reading
  - Sixth-grade level reader (6000–8500 words)
  - Use of primary reference materials encouraged
  - Literature and classics assigned

- Spelling and writing
  - More than 3000 words mastered
  - Original short stories, poems, compositions expected
  - More lengthy detailed reports and term projects

- Math
  - Division with 2-digit or 3-digit divisors
  - Simple algebraic expressions
  - Measurement, time, money skills mastered
  - Decimals and percentages

Assessment of Academic Skills

If a child is experiencing difficulties with school learning, the assessment of academic competencies and school function *begins* with obtaining information about the child's level of academic achievement. Is the child achieving on a level commensurate with expectations for age and grade level? Sources for verifying such information would include parental report, consultations with the child's teacher or school principal, school records and report cards concerning the child, and possibly referral for formal assessment through individually administered achievement tests. Such testing may be available on referral through the local school system. On occasion, it may be preferable to request achievement testing through an agency or clinic independent of the school system. Should there be a discrepancy between the child's measured level of academic achievement and age or grade level expectations in one or more of the basic subject areas, further investigation and assessment to help determine the reason for the discrepancy is definitely warranted. Review of the child's school history may reveal a checkered record of school attendance. Lengthy or frequent absences from school usually adversely affect school performance. Moves resulting in transfer from one school to another may contribute to setbacks and poor academic progress. Inadequate preparation for entering the school experience may account for some youngsters' extraordinary difficulties with acquiring language, learning to read, understanding numbers and developing quantitative skills, producing legible writing, or attending sufficiently well to learn in a standard classroom setting. Slow cognitive development or limited intellectual potential may underline a child's poor academic achievement. Previously undetected physical conditions—such as some degree of hearing impairment, visual defects, metabolic disorders—may account for a child's difficulties with learning. Factors such as investment, social adjustment, emotional maturity, family harmony, friendship networks, and attitude toward the value of school should also be explored as these may directly affect the child's performance in school.

If the presenting complaint includes problems with performance in school, the following questions should be considered:

- What is the child's school history (age at which school enrollment began, attendance record, any changes in school placement, promotions or retentions, disciplinary actions, parent–teacher conferences)?

- What is the child's academic achievement profile? Is the child demonstrating achievement commensurate with expectations for age and grade placement?
- Is there any reason to suspect specific learning disabilities?
- Suspect globally lower cognitive functioning? Intellectual brilliance?
- Suspect developmental delay or deviance?
- Are there physical conditions or medical concerns that may be contributing to or interfering with reported school performance?
- Are there social or emotional factors that may influence reported school performance?

Sources of information for addressing such questions would include:

- Parental interview
- Review of school records
- Phone contact or interview with school personnel (teacher, principal, guidance counselor, school nurse)
- Results from academic achievement testing
- Results from individually administered psychological and diagnostic educational testing
- Child interview

What is it that an educational specialist assesses when conducting an evaluation of a child's academic skills? Diagnostic tests of reading include measures of word recognition, decoding, and comprehension of written material. Auditory and visual perceptual skills and memory skills would also be assessed. Proficiency with both oral and silent readings—including reading rate, fluency, and phrasing—would be measured. Assessment of math or number skills might cover sequencing, seriation, memory, conservation, visual–spatial organization, numeration, reasoning skills, and computation skills. The application of math skills to concepts of time, measurement, and money, and to the solution of verbally presented problems also enters the comprehensive assessment of the child's ability to deal with numbers. Factors such as established handedness, type of pencil grasp, sitting posture, orientation of paper, letter formation, figure drawing, spacing, legibility, speed, and fluency enter the assessment of handwriting skills. Ability to recognize graphemes (letters and symbols), sequencing and memory skills, understanding of syllabication, and synthesis skills all enter the diagnostic evaluation of spelling—beyond demonstration of how many words a child can spell aloud or on paper. Throughout the evaluation of academic competencies, an astute evaluator will be observing for indications of learning style. Matching recommended instructional approaches, materials, and techniques to a particular child's demonstrated propensities or style of learning is the major contribution that an educational specialist can make.

Some of the more frequently used and popular measures of academic achievement that the clinician may encounter are highlighted in Table 2.

Maintaining successful performance in school is important not only to future life goals but also to the confirmation of self-worth and to the establishment of confidence in the growing child. Complaints about achievement and adjustment in school are common among those youngsters referred for mental health evaluations and services. Concerns about a child's school performance should be taken seriously and investigated through interviews, phone contacts, obtaining school records, and referral for formal evaluations where indicated. A significant discrepancy between a child's measured level of academic achievement and what is generally expected of students at the same age and grade level signals the need to refer for more elaborate and sophisticated diagnostic evaluation of the child's learning abilities and style.

ASSESSMENT OF VISUAL PERCEPTUAL MOTOR SKILLS

Assessment of perceptual motor skills comprises an area of specialized testing often conducted by trained psychologists. Development of adequate visual perceptual, visual memory, eye-hand, and integrative skills contributes to the child's com-

Table 2. Academic Achievement Tests and Diagnostic Tests of Educational Attainments

Test	Age/Grade	Description
Wide Range Achievement Test	5–adult K–post-12th	Brief screening measure of letter and word recognition, spelling and writing, and number and computational skills.
Peabody Individual Achievement Test	K–12th	Individually administered test of achievement in word recognition, reading comprehension, spelling, math, and general information.
Woodcock-Johnson Psychoeducational Battery	3–adult	Lengthy instrument containing multiple subtests designed to measure achievement in academic and basic learning skills.
Gray Oral Reading Test	1st–12th	Yields descriptive and diagnostic information about competency of oral reading skills.
Woodcock Reading Mastery Tests	K–12th	Contains five subjects: word identification, word comprehension, word attack, passage comprehension, and letter identification.
Spache Diagnostic Reading Scales	1st–8th	Individually administered test of oral reading, paragraph comprehension, word recognition, and decoding skills.
Durrell Analysis of Reading Difficulty	1st–6th	Lengthy assessment of skills necessary for competency with reading; contains 13 subtests.
KeyMath Diagnostic Arithmetic Test	preK–6th	Contains 14 subtests organized into 3 major areas of assessment: content (numeration, fractions, geometry, symbols), operations (addition, subtraction, multiplication, division, mental computation, numerical reasoning), and application (word problems, missing elements, money, measurement, time).
Morrison-McCall Spelling Test	1st–12th	Dictated spelling test that yields grade level score and records types of errors made.
Test of Written Spelling	1st–12th	Assesses both predictably (regular) spelled words and unpredictable spelling (nonregular) of words.

petency in learning and performing certain academic tasks (principally reading and writing). Deficits in these skills may reflect organically based learning disabilities or impairments. The ability to integrate visual and motor functions requires simultaneous processing of several stimuli and the smooth coordination of receptive, organizational, planning, and expressive capacities. Assessment of such skills, therefore, presumes to provide some reflection of the integrity of the central nervous system.

Assuming that visual acuity has been checked through an eye examination, visual perceptual skills constitute the first level of assessment. Accurate reception of visual image and interpretation of visually presented information should be tested under conditions that do not require a motor response. The child's responses to some of the items on the Wechsler scales may provide an indication of visual perceptual skills. A popular assessment tool is the *Motor-Free Visual Perception Test*. Portions of the *Detroit Tests of Learning Aptitude* (DTLA) may also be used to assess visual perceptual skills, visual memory, and visual–motor integration skills.

By far the most widely used tests of visual–motor capabilities are the *Visual Motor Gestalt Test* (Bender-Gestalt) and the VMI. The Bender-Gestalt has been in use clinically since the 1930s. It consists of nine classic geometric designs to be copied on paper. The accuracy of the child's efforts in drawing the figures, the organization of the figures on the paper, the size, the symmetry, and the formation are all considered in scoring and interpreting performance on this test. What the child reproduces can be used as an indicator of maturational level and may provide insight into possible organic dysfunctions. The VMI has been in use since the 1960s. Again, copying geometric designs on paper is required. However, the test consists of 24 figures arranged in ascending order of complexity reflecting a sequential development according to age level criteria. The test format is more highly structured on the VMI than on the Bender-Gestalt. Criteria for scoring children's performance are well delineated in the VMI test manual, which also contains suggestions for remedial procedures should results of testing indicate deficiencies.

Neither the Bender-Gestalt nor the VMI are timed. Contrasting a child's performance on timed versus untimed tasks can often yield interesting diagnostic information. One subtest of the DTLA involves demonstration of eye-hand speed and precision. Performance on the Coding or Digit Symbol subtests of the Wechsler scale may also be interpreted in light of speed and accuracy under timed conditions. Portions of some educational tests involve copying words, sentences, or symbols within given time constraints. Such tasks may prove useful as a practical measure of a child's ability to perform complex tasks requiring visual–motor integration skills under circumstances resembling conditions in a classroom.

CHILDREN'S DRAWINGS

Children's drawings have occupied an important place in the psychological testing battery. These easily administered tests are readily accepted by children. Drawing is a well-established route of communication with children. Materials (a pencil or crayons and some plain white paper) are of minimal cost and maximum availability in most settings.

Purposes of and Indications for Children's Drawings

- To begin a test battery as a means of establishing rapport with the child and putting the child at ease.
- To obtain a quick, rough, screening level estimate of personality-related concerns, fine motor control and visual–motor integration, skills, intelligence, and ability to attend to a task or details.
- To assess very young children or children with expressive language difficulties: drawings are relatively nonverbal and are not compromised or limited by the child's verbal expressive abilities.

Limitations of Children's Drawings

- The major limitation of drawings is when their use exceeds their screening level, rough estimate, hypothesis-generating capacities.

- The use of drawings is also limited by perceptual or fine motor handicapping conditions (e.g., children with severe neuromaturational delay or motor spasticity).

Varieties of Children's Drawings

The common varieties of drawings used and their interpretations are discussed below.

Human figure drawings (draw a person or draw a child) are generally administered individually, providing the child with a pencil, eraser, and plain white paper. Crayons are sometimes provided as a variation, but pens are rarely used. Instructions are generally kept simple, such as: "Please make me a drawing of a complete, whole child (or person)." Following the drawing of the child as a person, one variation is to request a drawing of the opposite-sexed child or person to the one first drawn. Another variation is to make an inquiry regarding the person/child drawn asking about his or her age, name, sex, person from real life it may resemble, and so on.

In the *house/tree/person test*, a child is asked to draw pictures of a house, a tree, and a person (in any order) on separate pieces of plain paper. The use of crayons for color is a popular variant. Interpretations of the drawings are derived through their study as displaced or "projected" self-referents. Interpretation takes into consideration the following:

- The "mood" suggested by the drawing.
- The implied competence and "stature."
- The age and sex portrayed relative to the age and sex of the child.
- Body parts that appear to be overemphasized or neglected relative to the portrayal in the rest of the drawing.
- Erasures or other evidence of confusion, distortion, or misrepresentation, a possible indication of anxiety regarding some part of the body and its perceived ability to function.
- General line quality—whether tentative, light, vague, dark, or pressured, or moderate and assured—a possible indication of self-esteem and self-assurance.

- Motor control, perceptual accuracy, distortion, and other signs of "organicity" or neuromaturational delay.

For a *kinetic family drawing*, the child is instructed: "For this drawing I would like you to draw a picture that includes everyone in your family doing something." If the child questions whether extended family should be included, it can be left to the child's discretion. If the child questions whether he or she should be included, the child's own inclination should be noted, but the child should be instructed to do so. If the child is not included in the drawing, that should be noted, but then the child should be instructed to include himself or herself. If the child asks whether the family should be doing something together or individually, the decision may be left to the child's discretion. The names, ages, sexes, and activities (if unclear) of all persons represented in the drawing should be recorded.

Interpretation of the family drawing is based, in part, on the consideration of the following elements:

- Who is included or omitted.
- The activities: whether engaged in together or individually, competitive or cooperative, their nature, and quality.
- Who is mutually engaged with whom, who is separated off, who is "involved," who is "distant."
- What alliances exist, either of a supportive or tension-producing nature.
- Relative "closeness" in family relations as represented by physical distance between family members, interactions, who's facing whom, who is physically cut-off from whom.
- Activities and person placement as an indication of perception of family roles vis-à-vis the child.

PROJECTIVE OR PERSONALITY-BASED ASSESSMENTS

Projective or personality-based psychological testing originated close in time to cognitive testing. Projective testing, although studied extensively and empirically validated, rests on one basic theoretical principle: that given a sufficiently ambiguous stimulus, a subject's response will be the result of his or her own projected personality. Expressed another way, the picture reveals the nature of the artist; the story reveals the nature of the author; the percept reveals the nature of the perceiver. Thus children, in their responses to ambiguous but standardized test stimuli, can reveal to the trained observer needs, concerns, coping styles, ability to integrate and tolerate affect, capacity to test reality, and perceptions of oneself and others.

Purpose and Indications for Projective Testing

- Projective testing may be useful as another piece of independent data (apart from history, mental status, play interview) in the differential diagnosis of psychiatric problems. This is particularly true in complex situations in which it is otherwise difficult to assign weights to various factors or diagnostic data being observed or being reported.
- Major psychopathology, including thought disorder, affective disorder, or other psychiatric disorders, is usually revealed through projective instruments.
- Projective tests can help in the assessment of suicidal risk and other impulse disorders: how pressing and conscious the concerns and ideation are and how they relate to other aspects of personality functioning.
- Projective tests may provide a perspective on overall personality functioning: coping and defensive styles, adequacy of defenses, strength of various affects, integration of affect, and frightening thoughts or affects being defended.
- Projective tests may help clarify a child's self-perception and perception of significant others, whether the perception is conscious or not.
- "Opening up" an otherwise verbally or behaviorally constricted child may result from projective tests. These tests may function as a "window" on personality and psychological functioning when other avenues appear closed.
- The relative role of affective or emotional factors in other behavioral concerns, symptoms, academic problems or peer/socialization difficulties can be assessed.

- Projective testing may be "politically" helpful in justifying (e.g., courts or educational boards) special needs or residential therapeutic placement.

Limitations of Projective Testing

- Children must voluntarily participate and cooperate to a maximum extent for the testing to yield useful data. In the case of flat refusals to participate, no data can be obtained.
- A child with extreme emotional constriction or severely impaired relatedness would yield data of dubious quality or validity.
- Projective testing is not fully independent of verbal expressive abilities, which places limits on its usefulness under the following conditions:
  - Extremely young children with no or very limited language skills or abilities.
  - Moderately to severely retarded children with limited language skills or abilities.
  - Children with major expressive language problems; any results with such classes of children, if possible at all, would require careful, qualified interpretation.

- Projective testing may be experienced as anxiety-arousing to some children. In actuality, this would be true of only a small minority and would more likely affect older adolescents than younger children.
- Results are likely to be inadequate if tests are given, scored, or interpreted by other than a qualified professional pathologist.
- Cost may be a limiting factor. Projective tests require time to administer, score, interpret, and write up. Insurance, ability to pay, and its necessity must be carefully considered and weighed.

Types of Projective Testing and Possible Interpretations

There are many classes of projective tests; the major ones are discussed below. These tests tend to vary in: (a) the age of the child for which it is appropriately given, (b) the degree of structure or ambiguity of the test stimuli, (c) the types or areas of information that are specifically elicited, and (d) the specific kinds of interpretations that can potentially be made.

Drawings. Children's drawings were discussed earlier in this chapter. As projective tests, they tend to have particularly rich potential to tap self-related concerns such as self-esteem and body image. Family perceptions, relations, and role perceptions are also revealed. As projective tests, children's drawings are a rich source of hypothesis, but absolute interpretations are difficult and rest on corroborating data obtained elsewhere in the test battery.

Incomplete Sentence Tests. There are many forms of child and adolescent incomplete sentence tests. Among the most popular is The Rotter Incomplete Sentences Blank. In all versions, the child is asked to complete a list of sentence stems that have no endings. Examples might be "Howard was sorry after he . . .," "Ray thought that his mother should . . .," or "Phillip felt that his future. . . ." Responses are checked for themes, sequencing of material, and unusual or unique sentence endings.

Incomplete sentence tests are helpful in learning the following kinds of information:

- Indications of stresses, pressures, needs;
- More conscious emotional concerns;
- Worries, fears, anxieties;
- Additional self- and family-related perceptions;
- General indication of reality testing and orientation, and
- Some indication of affective pulls, coping styles, and typically utilized defenses.

Rorschach (Inkblot Test). The Rorschach has been used with children of all ages, adolescents, and adults. The test plates or inkblots are the same in all cases; however, the administration (to some extent) and interpretation (to a larger extent) vary depending on the person's age. This test is generally not administered to children under the age of 4 or 5. The Rorschach uses the least structured and most ambiguous projective test stimuli available. It consists of ten cards presented serially. These cards vary in black and white versus color content as well as form ambiguity. The child is instructed to look at the cards and describe what they resemble. Responses and behavior are carefully recorded. One or sometimes two detailed inquiries regarding the initial percepts are necessary to complete scoring and interpretation.

The Rorschach yields the following kinds of information:

- Reality testing, accuracy, orientation, and adequacy under various emotional conditions;
- Defenses, their uses and adequacy;
- Ability to handle and integrate affect;
- Presence of strong affect states and how they may be experienced;
- Indications of suicidality;
- Object relations: orientation and receptivity to interpersonal relations; and
- Creativity, emotional resourcefulness, and ability to integrate affect and cognition.

Thematic Apperception Test (TAT) and Children's Apperception Test (CAT). Apperception tests are a standard part of most projective batteries. The CAT is used most often with children from age 3 to 7 whereas the TAT is used from age 8 on up. The CAT is composed of 10 cards depicting various younger animal-figures engaged in a variety of activities with adult counterparts. Pictured themes include nurturance, family competition, sibling rivalry, socialization, toilet training, and handling of aggression.

The TAT is comprised of a wide variety of cards to be used by men, women, boys, or girls. The psychologist is free to choose (usually 10) cards that have thematic material of greater relevance to the case. Cards are drawings that depict children and adults in various poses, activities, interactions, and postures. Themes run a gamut of affective states and interpersonal dilemmas. However, the drawings are sufficiently ambiguous to have a wide variety of perceptions possible on any given card.

For both apperception tests, the child is generally instructed to tell a story from his or her own imagination, using the card as a stimulus. If not included spontaneously in the story offered, the tester may inquire about perceptions regarding what is happening in the story, who the various characters might be, what each of the characters is thinking or feeling, and what would happen next or be the ending of the story.

A wide range of interpretations regarding reality perceptions, coping styles, affective stresses, and perception of oneself and significant others is potentially available in the scoring or analysis of apperception test responses. Apperception tests provide corroborating evidence from a range of other tests such as drawings, sentence completions, and the Rorschach. Since they are somewhat more structured than the Rorschach, they are not as sensitive to reality distortion potential or less conscious issues and material. However, responses to these tests may suggest potential for emotional functioning under more favorable, more clearly structured situations and environments.

Other Projective Tests. A number of other, less frequently used, projective tests are available for children and adolescents. Among them are the Education Apperception Test, which assesses adjustment to specific educational environment situations, and the Blacky Pictures, an older picture test for children that attempts to assess psychosexual development. New projective tests appear in research and are occasionally published when research is favorable. An example of a new test is the Roberts Apperception Test for children, which attempts to assess adjustment to more contemporary interpersonal events in children's lives.

However, the Tasks of Emotional Development Test (TED) may be the most popular "other" projective test. It consists of 12 cards depicting photographs of children and adults in various situations or problem confrontations. Separate sets of cards exist for latency-aged boys and girls, as well as adolescent boys and girls. Similar to the apperception tests, children are asked to make up a story about what is happening. Children's responses to the TED allow for the detection of areas of specific concern in psychological developmental tasks, reality distortions, affective pressures, coping styles, and self/other perceptions. However, the cards favor the perception of feelings for and expectations regarding the specific tasks of:

- Peer socialization,
- Parental nurturance,
- Peer aggression,
- School achievement,
- Conscience and impulse control,
- Separating from parents,
- Sex role identification,
- Sibling rivalry,
- Accepting limits from parents,
- Handling parental intimacy,
- Conflict resolution with parents, and
- Developing a self-identity.

Empirical/Objective Personality Measures. Empirical or objective personality measures are generally used less often with children as opposed to adults. These tests are generally in the form of a long list of true/false or yes/no answers. Scoring is objective in that one's pattern of responses is compared with that of groups of "known" type. Normative data is derived through strict empirical data collection. Scoring of such tests is often done by computer and yields a computerized "personality profile."

The Minnesota Multiphasic Personality Inventory is the best known and most widely used of such tests. It is composed of over 500 true/false questions. Norms have been developed for adolescents to whom the test may be administered. There are no "child" norms; this test is not used with preadolescents. When appropriate and valid, scoring will yield a personality profile as well as an indication of how high or low an individual scores (above, below, or within normal limits) on a number of scales. These include hypochondriasis, depression, hysteria, psychopathic deviate, masculinity/femininity, paranoia, psychasthenia, schizophrenia, mania, and social introversion.

Another similar objective measure growing in popularity in research and clinical use is the Personality Inventory for Children. In this test, it is the *parent* who responds to a list of 600 true/false questions regarding perceptions of the child. Profiles and state scores falling within or outside of "normal" limits have been developed, including, for example, depression, self-concept, anxiety, reality distortion, peer relations, conscience development, activity level, somatic complaints, school adjustment, and family discord.

A final, related instrument, the Vineland Adaptive Behavior Scales (a recent revision of the older Vineland Social Maturity Scale) exists in three versions to assess adaptive behaviors, strengths, and weaknesses in children from birth to 19 years of age. They are: (a) a Survey Form for screening, placement, and diagnostic purposes; (b) an Expanded Form for developing specific educational or treatment plans; and (c) a Classroom Edition. In all forms, a semistructured 30- to 60-minute interview is administered to parents or primary caregivers. Scores, normed with percentile ranks, are available in the following adaptive domains: communication, daily living skills, socializations, motor skills, and an adaptive behavior composite.

Conclusion

Interpretation of data gained in projective or personality-based assessments is a complex art and science at present. Therefore, conclusions are best drawn with consultation of an appropriately trained professional.

NEUROPSYCHOLOGICAL TESTING

Neuropsychological testing is a specialized field of testing requiring specific training of the psychologist that is often beyond the scope of standard clinical training. It is similar to other forms of neurodiagnostic evaluation in its endeavor to permit accurate references regarding the size, location, and processes involved in different types of brain lesions and dysfunctions. However, although it focuses on the direct appraisal of adaptive functions and abilities, it may provide detailed specialization of the behavioral effects of brain impairment. Neuropsychological testing may be used to devise an appropriate plan of rehabilitation of an individual's particular pattern of spared/impaired abilities.

Purposes and Indications of Neuropsychological Testing

Child clinical neuropsychology has been defined as the application of psychological and neuropsychological knowledge to the assessment and treatment of children and adolescents having neurological disorders. Neuropsychological testing attempts to assess the psychological and behavioral sequelae of such illnesses. Assessment may range from commonly described deficits in intellectual-cognitive functions, memory, and sensorimotor functions to those less frequently thought of as related to injury or disease, such as deficits in social adjustment and perspective, social skills, personality characteristics, or goal-directed behavior.

Adult and child neuropsychologists' tasks differ in relation to the nature of diseases affecting children vis-à-vis adults. Adult neuropsychologists are more likely to reassess functioning of individuals affected by alcoholism, multiple sclerosis, Alzheimer's disease, and cerebral-vascular accidents. In contrast, child neuropsychologists are more likely to evaluate children with Reye's syndrome, subacute sclerosing panencephalitis, and *Haemophilus influenzae* meningitis. Child neuropsychologists are clearly expanding into the study and clinical assessment of children with learning disabilities, head trauma, tumors, Tourette's syndrome, brain infections, and congenital and biological compromises.

Historically, clinical neuropsychology has emphasized the development and standardization of neuropsychological test batteries that have incorporated "tried and true" cognitive tests, educational tests, and visual–motor tests (previously described) as well as adding specifically focused newly developed tests. Recent trends in neuropsychological testing include behavioral assessment with behavioral treatment techniques, where applicable.

In summary, neuropsychological testing may be helpful in evaluating the spared or impaired psychological functions of children affected by *specific* or *suspected neurological disease*. In some cases, these can lead to specific behavioral treatment recommendations that follow from the pattern of strengths and weaknesses revealed.

Limitations of Neuropsychological Testing

Child neuropsychological assessment remains a relatively young subspecialty. Although alive with active and current research, the field has not reached a level of full maturity, at this time, equivalent to adult neuropsychology.

Child neuropsychology and child neuropsychological assessment is limited by certain factors inherent in the developing organism. First, a child's nervous system is in a constant state of change due to factors such as continuing growth, myelination, and innervation. This state of flux places limits on the interpretation of data for predictive purposes. Further, the effect of neurologic damage may produce vastly different cognitive and behavioral sequelae in a child who has not yet acquired skills as compared to an adult whose skills were previously established. The response of the yet "plastic" nervous system for predictive purposes also remains uncertain.

Types of Neuropsychological Tests

There are two main neuropsychological test batteries used in the assessment of children:

Halstead-Reitan Neuropsychological Battery. This battery of tests has been shown to distinguish accurately between normal youngsters and those from variously composed groups with confirmed brain damage. Children appropriate for testing range in age from 5 to 14 years old. Comparative results have been reported for children with minimal cerebral dysfunction, mental retardation, and learning disabilities.

A neuropsychological assessment with this battery will universally include WISC-R and an educational achievement test. Specific to the Halstead-Reitan battery would be some of the following neuropsychological tests:

- A category test to assess complex concept formation and abstraction skills.
- Tactual performance test to assess tactile form discrimination, kinesthesis, and manual dexterity.
- Speech sounds perception test to assess the ability to perceive the spoken stimulus-sound through hearing and to relate the perception through vision to a correct configuration of letters on a test form.
- Marching test to assess gross skeletal muscular function.
- Finger-tapping test to assess digit dexterity and left–right-sided strength comparisons.
- Color form test to assess organizational ability.
- Progressive figure test (a more difficult version of Color form test).
- Matching pictures test to assess simple abstraction and concept formation.

Luria-Nebraska Neuropsychological Battery (Children's Revision). This battery appears to be gaining an unusual amount of recent acceptance as a new psychological test instrument. Its use, however, is restricted to children in the limited age range of 8 to 12 years. The battery consists of 149 items that are grouped into 11 summary scales:

- Motor: fine motor speed, coordination, control
- Rhythm: discrimination, reproduction of patterns
- Tactile: sensitivity to localized stimuli
- Visual: visual recognition and use of spatial relationships
- Receptive speech: discriminating sounds and understanding language
- Expressive language: initiating verbal responses
- Writing: copy, spell, write
- Reading: letters, words, sentences, paragraphs

- Arithmetic: mathematical concepts and processes
- Memory: verbal and nonverbal
- Intellectual processes: ability to make simple generalized and basic deductions

Interpretations are made in the synthesis and assessment of patterns of strengths and weaknesses revealed in the test scores. Batteries can be used to assess the presence or absence of probable neurological impairment through the use of empirically derived cut-off scores that divide children that age "within normal limits" from those outside of normal limits. Thus a diagnosis of impaired or unimpaired may be made on the basis of quantitative, objective scores.

Finer interpretations are made from the exact nature of the pattern or scores achieved on the specific battery subtests. Strengths and weaknesses provide a description of functions that a child processes to learn and apply general skills. Weak areas may require remediation or treatment where feasible. Strengths may often be used to offset or circumvent weakened or impaired areas of functioning.

References

1. Wide Range Achievement Test (available from Jastak Associates, Inc., 1526 Gilpin Avenue, Wilmington, Delaware 19806), 1978

2. Groth-Marnat G: Handbook of Psychological Assessment. New York, Van Nostrand Reinhold, 1984

3. Tramontana MG: Neuropsychological evaluation in child/adolescent psychiatric disorders: current status. The Psychiatric Hospital 14:158–162, 1983

4. Sparrow S, Balla D, Cicchetti D: The Vineland Adaptive Behavior Scale: Interview Edition, Survey Form. Circle Pines, Minn, American Guidance Service, 1984 (This screening test is not currently in widespread clinical practice because it is newly designed and requires both application and sustained clinical exposure.)

Appendix 1: Cognitive Screening of the Grade School Child

P. S. B. Sarma, M.B., B.S.

Cognitive dysfunctions constitute the essential criteria for some childhood diagnoses from the *Diagnostic and Statistical Manual of Mental Disorders, Third Edition (DSM-III)* (mental retardation and certain specific developmental disorders). Cognitive dysfunctions are also associated with other diagnostic categories and may either be the result of the disorder (e.g., depression) or may be implicated in aggravating the severity of the disorder (e.g., attention deficit disorder with hyperactivity, conduct disorders, separation anxiety disorder). Hence it is important that the comprehensive psychiatric evaluation of an elementary school child include consideration of cognitive function. Although standardized psychological and achievement testing is the optimal means of accomplishing this task, it requires the involvement of another mental health professional and the associated procedural complexities. Particularly when we are asked to see a child in consultation on the pediatric floor or in the clinic, it is very helpful to have a way of doing a reliable and brief cognitive screening. The most common areas of dysfunctions are in the ability to deal with written language and in the ability to deal with number concepts. The procedure described below is part of the Brief Intellectual Screening Test for Elementary-Grade Children (BISTEC), which was developed by the author. It requires no more than 10 minutes and incorporates skills that are exhibited by the average child between the ages of 5 and 11.

Any child who manifests a lag of more than 1 year between expected performance for age and actual performance is in need of more extensive testing. BISTEC quotient in reading, spelling, and arithmetic can be calculated as follows:

$$\text{BISTEC Q} = \frac{\text{Mental Age}}{\text{Chronological Age}} \times 100$$

In a sample of children ranging in age from 5 to 11, the following correlations between BISTEC quotients and the corresponding standard scores in the Wide Range Achievement Test were obtained: reading ($N = 54$), 0.86 ($p < .001$); spelling ($N = 116$), 0.83 ($p < .001$); and arithmetic ($N = 116$), 0.83 ($p < .001$). In a sample of 31 children who were retested after an average interval of 2 months, the BISTEC quotient scores obtained a Pearson product moment correlation of 0.64 in arithmetic, 0.89 in spelling, and 0.93 in reading.

Spelling

The spelling test is given before the reading test because some of the items are shared. Furthermore, if the child is able to spell at a level of 9 years or higher, the reading test need not be administered.

The child is first asked to name the items on the sheet. If the child has difficulty, he or she is told what the items are. Then the child is asked to print the word under each item, starting with "cat." After the item "book" the child is asked to spell "read." We can stop when the child makes mistakes with three consecutive words. If the child seems hesitant with any item, the child is encouraged to guess the spelling even if he or she does not know it.

Scoring. We start with the base age of 6 and give a credit of 4 months each for the correctly spelled words "cat, dog, and man" and a credit of 6 months each for the words "bird, horse, book, read, circle, square, diamond, and cross."

Reading

This is administered if the child's spelling skills are below 9 years of age.

Scoring. Starting with a base age of 4½ years, a credit of 1 month each is given for the six letters and six numbers. The words "clown, school, began, wanted, and after" are given 4 months credit each.

Arithmetic

A child who is 6 years or older is given the sheet with the arithmetic items and asked to do as many items as he or she can. The child is stopped at the end of 5 minutes. If the child is finished before the 5 minutes are up, the items that are incorrect are pointed out and the child is allowed to correct as many as he or she wants within the 5 minutes time. If the child is unable to do more than two of the written items correctly, the verbal items are administered.

Scoring. Starting with a base age of 5 years, verbal items are given 4 months credit each. If only written items are administered, the scoring starts with a base age of 6 years and each correctly answered item is given a credit of 4 months.

The above procedure is applicable only to those children who are reared in English-speaking families in the United States and who attend accredited schools. Any child who appears to be functioning at a level that is 1 year or more below his or her chronological age in any area should be evaluated with an appropriate psychological battery.

Chapter 5

Formulation, Differential Diagnosis, and Treatment Planning

Kenneth S. Robson, M.D.

FORMULATION

In child psychiatric assessments, even more than in general psychiatry, sufficient data to make a definitive diagnosis may only become available with the passage of time. This is the case in part because of the diagnostician's need for extensive exposure to both child and family and for the establishment of trust. Sexual abuse, for example, may be suspected but undocumented for long periods of time. In addition, the nature of childhood and development is such that the evolution of certain pathologic conditions, the transformation of one condition "into" a second, or the disappearance of less grave disorders can require months or years. Furthermore, the plasticity and lack of differentiation in the young child (5 years old and under) makes the discrimination between normal and pathologic behaviors, between "phenotype and genotype," more difficult to assess. Sleep disturbances in 3-year-olds are to be expected; in 10-year-olds they may be part of a major depression or dysthymic disorder. Tantrums in the 2-year-old are normative; in the 12-year-old they can herald the onset of more major mental illness. In many respects, then, diagnosis in child psychiatry is a longitudinal process.

Nevertheless, one cannot wait for time to pass. The establishment of a working formulation is essential for therapeutic interventions to begin. The formulation should not be confused with diagnosis and is concerned with: (a) life events and chronology, as they relate to the emergence of psychopathology; (b) the pathophysiology of the symptoms, signs, and behaviors in question (see Chapter 1), and (c) the current physical and developmental status of the child (using Erikson and A. Freud).

The formulation is a kind of road map for the diagnostician and therapist. By pulling together the data gathered in the evaluation, it forces the clinician to integrate findings, generate clinical hypotheses, and plan thoughtfully for interventions. A well-developed formulation should lead to more definitive differential diagnoses as well. In another sense the formulation represents a "distillate" of the data, a concise crystallization of the essential facts, events, and processes at the center of the child's difficulties. In life not too much can go wrong if a child is genuinely loved, in good health, and in reasonably secure reality circumstances. A well-executed formulation should require a paragraph in written reports and 5 minutes in spoken presentations.

DIFFERENTIAL DIAGNOSIS

The history of systems of diagnostic classification in child psychiatry is of interest in its own right (1). The shifting theoretical models of the field can be traced through its nosologies. Each of these systems is out of synchrony with certain clinical syndromes. The Group for the Advancement of Psychiatry classification (1), although currently out of favor, is clinically useful and emphasizes developmental and pathophysiologic aspects of the child; their monograph is well worth reading, keeping in mind that its primary orientation is psychodynamic. This system deals more effectively than the *Diagnostic and Statistical Manual of Mental Disorders, Third Edition (DSM-III)*

(2), in most respects, with less serious developmental disorders, reactive states, and certain character or personality types met with in childhood.

On the other hand, the system now in use, *DSM-III*, has powerful descriptive reliability; the orientation is clearly medical. Because of such a perspective, this system tends to be more applicable to the severe disorders of childhood and adolescence that have a structure to some degree fixed. Developmental crises and deviations, reactive conditions, and familial dysfunction fit with greater difficulty into *DSM-III*, whereas autism, schizophrenia, and affective disorders are well considered. Nevertheless, this multi-axial system approximates the medical model and is vigorously designed and field-tested. *It should be used with every child.* The compact paperbound mini-version of *DSM-III* belongs in every diagnostician's desk (3).

Diagnostic categories will relate in varying degrees to the formulation. The exercise of differential diagnosis, however, is essential and invaluable to the clinician. Acknowledging that diagnosis is at best an *approximation*, contains only partial truths and incomplete data, may not point back to etiology or forward to treatment planning, and is at times illusory, it still serves several important ends: (a) clarity and rigor of clinical thinking, (b) problem-oriented treatment planning, (c) standardization for purposes of reporting and research, and (d) compatibility with the medical model and tradition. In addition, there is the issue of third-party reimbursement. With increasing scrutiny by regulatory bodies, fixed limits on hospital and ambulatory levels of payment for clinical services, and the introduction of diagnosis-related groups that establish length of stay in hospitals, the utilization of diagnostic categories (as developed in *DSM-III*) is mandatory.

To avoid the often false reassurance of diagnostic labels, the child psychiatrist is advised to utilize *both* formulation and differential diagnoses in arriving at a treatment plan. In a sense, the formulation is related more closely to function and the diagnoses to structure. By using both perspectives, more reliably designed interventions will take place. For example, attention deficit disorder is a favorite diagnosis in many child psychiatric centers. The criteria for diagnosis of this condition in *DSM-III* are unambiguous. Unfortunately, impulsivity, hyperactivity, and attentional difficulties are common to many underlying clinical phenomena, such as anxiety, depression, pre-psychotic states, and neurointegrative deficits. Each of these phenomena may require specific therapeutic measures quite different from one another. Furthermore, the roles of familial dysfunction, empathic deficits, and overstimulation in the environment are addressed in the formulation, not the diagnosis, of attention deficit disorder. Hence, the wisdom of a combined approach that uses both data bases becomes clear.

TREATMENT PLANNING

With both formulation and differential diagnoses in mind, the clinician is in a position to design an initial treatment plan. As noted in Chapter 2, the optimal plan in contrast to the possible plan may be discrepant in major ways. In particular, the limitations of the family's (or institution's) psychological *and* fiscal resources will limit the child psychiatrist's recommendations and freedom of therapeutic movement. Like politics, treatment planning is the "art of the possible." Although these realities are sometimes (if not often) discouraging, at the same time creative efforts are called into play; necessity can serve as the parent of therapeutic invention. Furthermore, there are few therapeutic outcome studies in child psychiatry that would support, with hard data, traditional or specific treatment regimens. Finally, more treatment is not necessarily better treatment. The physician in training will profit from an approach that is characterized by flexibility, curiosity, and a willingness to question traditional modes with a keen and observing eye. With these thoughts in mind, certain principles of therapeutic planning may be outlined:

- The *primary* goal of any therapeutic plan, regardless of the modalities involved, is developmental facilitation of the child.
- The biological family, or parties in loco parentis, must be

able to accept minimal essential aspects of this goal; one cannot treat most children or adolescents without significant collaboration from the parties involved, no matter how crucial the need. Hence, the decision *not* to treat should be appropriately exercised and may, in itself, be therapeutic.
- Financial resources necessary for any treatment plan—whether private, third party, or state/local—must be realistically assessed both before and in the context of planning. Available monies are the "bottom line" of therapeutic strategies.
- The child psychiatrist as treatment planner must be willing to assume a variety of roles that include psychotherapist; family worker; consultant to schools, courts, and social service agencies; child advocate in the political systems (e.g., schools, courts, summer camps) surrounding the child; and coordinator and choreographer of all of these.
- Multiple modalities of intervention are generally necessary. The therapeutic needs in any clinical situation *change*, however, with the passage of time, altered developmental status, improvement or deterioration in the child, and the availability of new resources. Regular reassessment of the original plan is essential.

COMMUNICATING DIAGNOSTIC INFORMATION AND TREATMENT PLANNING

The data from psychiatric evaluations and the treatment plans evolving from them are only as valuable as the skill with which they are conveyed to the key parties involved. Children, and in most instances, adolescents, are captive patients who do not refer themselves and cannot be treated without the support of parents, parties in loco parentis, referring nonpsychiatric physicians, and so on. Hence this critical juncture in the clinical process often requires exquisitely sensitive and tactful effort.

Whenever possible, sessions to review diagnostic issues and treatment considerations should include both parents. Children and adolescents can be given a choice to participate in some or all of the meeting, depending on clinical judgment and circumstances. With adolescents it is sometimes advisable to begin treatment *before* conveying further information to parents but to schedule this event at some point in the therapy. With children in foster care or institutional settings, choosing the appropriate participants may be more difficult; knowledge of the power structure and politics of the situation are essential.

Many diagnostic evaluations spontaneously establish both effective alliances with child and family and the need for ongoing treatment. When such is the case, the clinician's task is simply to maintain existing momentum. In other instances, however, parental anxiety, defensiveness, or outright hostility complicate matters and one walks a kind of therapeutic tightrope. There are no easy guidelines in the latter situation, although bluntness is best avoided unless essential. Further, parents need not hear a *DSM-III* diagnosis to feel satisfied that they know the facts. It is always important to stress a child's strengths and assets, as well as parents' commitment to parenting. At the same time, the clinician must convey the nature and quality of a child's difficulties in a manner that is thorough, convincing, and clearly understood. Using parents' own words and perceptions of their child is an appropriate starting point. "Nervous" may be preferred to "anxious," "problems with self-control" to "impulsive," "difficulty telling real from imaginary" to "psychotic" or "poor reality testing." Further, it is probably best to avoid predictions of prognosis or length of treatment unless necessary; these issues will become apparent in time or be more easily discussed when treatment has begun and parents can more readily accept serious disorders.

In conveying to parents the necessity for treatment, it is useful to be concrete. Discussion of *impairments in school functioning, personal relationships, level of unhappiness*, or *symptomatology* helps parents understand the deficits that a child experiences without undue guilt. To the inevitable question "what have we done to cause these problems" it can be helpful to point out that no psychiatric problem is caused by one source of difficulty; that genetic endowment, constitution and temperament, traumatic events and so on all play a role in the evolution of symptomatology. Finally, in certain situations, it may also be helpful to acknowledge with parents that they have a more difficult child who makes the job of parenting harder; such is often the case. If therapeutic interventions are refused but are, in the clinician's opinion, essential to avoid further deterioration or suicidal risk, directness and firmness are indicated. Confrontation and toughness in the face of necessity are valuable tools appropriate to the child psychiatrist's armamentarium.

Written materials deserve careful attention before they are sent on to parents, referral sources (including nonpsychiatric physicians), schools, and courts. A guiding principle is to say *as little* as possible in the *simplest* manner to convey the *essential* information for the party in question to know. Once written materials are sent out they become public information to most or all parties involved. One should not assume that all physician colleagues are psychiatrically sophisticated or sensitive to such issues as timing, terminology, and parental defensiveness. Collaborative editing with colleagues, such as clinical psychologists who have administered test protocols, is important and useful. Finally, in an era where hair-trigger litigation is epidemic, the child psychiatrist must consider the legal hazard of written clinical materials about highly sensitive matters including physical and sexual abuse, rape, abortion, drug abuse, criminal behavior, marital infidelity, and family "secrets." The clinician is advised to utilize care and tact and *always* preface sensitive issues with "reported" or "alleged" (e.g., abuse, neglect) in order to protect himself or herself, the clinician's institution, and, in some cases, the child and family members.

References

1. Group for the Advancement of Psychiatry: Psychopathological Disorders in Childhood: Theoretical Considerations and a Proposed Classification. New York, Group for the Advancement of Psychiatry, 1966

2. American Psychiatric Association: Diagnostic and Statistical Manual of Mental Disorders, Third Edition. Washington, DC, American Psychiatric Association, 1980
3. American Psychiatric Association: Quick Reference to the Diagnostic Criteria from DSM-III. Washington, DC, American Psychiatric Association, 1980

PART 2
APPROACHES TO TREATMENT

Chapter 6.	Introduction to Treatment	113
Chapter 7.	Therapeutics I: The Psychotherapies	119
Chapter 8.	Therapeutics II: Intensive Milieu Therapy, Behavior Therapy, and Hypnosis	131
Chapter 9.	Therapeutics III: Pharmacotherapy	149
Chapter 10.	Emergencies I	185
Chapter 11.	Emergencies II: Sexual Abuse and Rape in Childhood	213

Chapter 6

Introduction to Treatment

Kenneth S. Robson, M.D.

In Part 1 of this manual, a model of the pathophysiology of childhood disorders was presented (see Chapter 1). This model emphasizes the role of both internal and external overstimulation through excessive or insufficient, unmodulated levels of arousal-producing contact and empathic failures in parenting in creating a pathogenic environment and developmental deviance. Although far from exhaustive in accounting for pathologic conditions in childhood, this point of view appears to address a significant amount of variance in most clinical conditions and leads to concrete and practical approaches to therapeutic interventions, regardless of modality. Furthermore, although the degree of "fixed" or "structural" psychopathology is difficult to assess in most syndromes and symptom complexes (other than in the catastrophic disorders such as autism and schizophrenia), the model presented here focuses on the modifiable aspects of pathogenic conditions. Percentage-wise, in general, external overstimulation and empathic failures in parenting, through their accessibility to the clinician, offer the most powerful options for therapeutic influence. It follows, from this position, that therapeutic efforts directed at specific current dysfunctions in the parent or parent-surrogate environment are seen as most likely to produce change. Conversely, clinical energies directed toward the intrusive pathologic phenomena in the individual child are viewed as important but less relevant than environmental modifications in successful therapeutic outcomes.

Within the model espoused here, the goals of all forms of treatment remain the same: to modulate internal and external levels of stimulation impinging on the child and to increase empathic levels of caretaking in order to facilitate development. Hence, the psychoactive agent that reduces agitation, lowers levels of anxiety, or diminishes flooding of the child's ego with depressive affect can play a critical role in helping a child decrease internal levels of overstimulation or excessive vulnerability to external stimuli. Helping parents to relinquish seductive, "orgiastic" models of relatedness, or to avoid loss of impulse control with the child, and to remain related to the child rather than withdrawing in cold, destructive anger are commonly encountered strategies in modulating levels of parental overstimulation. For example, assisting the parent who views excessive masturbation in the prepubertal child as "being oversexed" to see such behavior as a reaction to isolation, depression, and separation concerns can convert unempathic, punitive, parental withdrawal to a comforting, supportive presence. Such shifts have great importance therapeutically. Again, the "crystals" of development require calm or even silence to take shape, and they are fractured by flooding.

The examples cited above convey the central thrust of the therapeutic model being described. Although the underlying concepts are relatively simple, they can be used to organize sensible, well-thought-out, and achievable therapeutic plans. Further, these same concepts provide ongoing evidence, a kind of "therapeutic gyroscope," to the child psychiatrist in his or her therapeutic "posture" with child, parents, schools, and courts. In Figure 1 this therapeutic schema is illustrated. Comparing Figure 1 with Chapter 1, Figure 2 will clarify the relationship between the pathophysiology of childhood disorders and corrective treatment strategies. Finally, because careful research into the process and outcome of child ther-

Introduction to Treatment 115

MODULATION OF OVERSTIMULATION

INTERNAL (CHILD)

- Gain self-control
- Reduce impulsiveness
- Stabilize regulation of self-esteem
- Decrease cathexis and ego-syntonicity of "orgiastic" mode
- Reduce vulnerability to anxiety
- Reduce depression
- Enhance all "ego" skills (e.g., learning, sports, peer relations)
- Diminish fears
- Strengthen reality testing
- Soften harsh and rigid self-criticism
- Use of psychoactive agents
- Reduce narcissistic "entitlement"
- Therapists' "ego-relatedness" with child

EXTERNAL (PARENTS)

- Encourage physical modesty
- Close bathroom and bedroom doors
- Have child sleep in own bed
- Avoid harsh, excessive, and frightening physical punishment
- Modulate and desexualize physical contact
- Increase parental "ego-relatedness"
- Increase parental "availability" by modifying depression, anxiety, and schizoid withdrawal
- Psychoactive drug treatment of appropriate symptoms and conditions
- Encourage interactions in play and games that soothe rather than excite
- Help child develop the capacity to be alone
- Separate from child in appropriate ways
- Substitution of alternative environment when necessary (foster care, residential)
- Consultation to school environment

INCREASED EMPATHIC CARETAKING

- Appreciation of meaning of child's behavior
- Appreciation of one's own behavior
- Institution of age-appropriate expectations with child
- Reduce need for child as "sustaining object"
- Help parents recall own childhood
- Acceptance of child's development as painful loss
- Reduce misperceptions of child's behavior and responses
- Enhance parental capacity to identify child's inner affective states
- Enhance parental capacity to identify own affective states
- Consultation to teachers
- Consultation to foster-parents, institutional staff
- Therapists' empathic relationships with child

FACILITATION OF CHILD'S DEVELOPMENT

apies is sparse, child psychiatry fellows are advised to read other thoughtful reviews of this subject (1).

GOALS AND MODELS OF TREATMENT

Although the larger goal of any therapeutic intervention—facilitation of the child's development—is evident, the process of clearly articulating *specific component goals* can facilitate cost-effective clinical work. Common examples include the following:

- Establishing a working alliance,
- Completing diagnostic evaluations,
- Starting psychoactive drugs,
- Establishing contact with school personnel,
- Returning a reluctant child to school,
- Resolving a crisis situation,
- Manipulating the environment,
- Advising lawyers and parents vis-à-vis disruptive custodial arrangements,
- Helping parents into individual or marital therapies,
- Helping child establish peer relationships, and
- Making ego-syntonic behaviors ego-alien.

Obviously, the nature of therapeutic goals will vary with the passage of time, developmental progress, and changing needs of the child and family. Winnicott's concept of the "holding environment" is applicable here. The therapist attempts to create an optimal environment, through all available means, within which healthy development can proceed.

Other critical variables over which one has little or no control will play a major role in the design feasibility of treatment interventions. For this reason, the therapist is advised to *prioritize goals* insofar as that is possible. Factors affecting treatment implementation include the following:

- The family's readiness for therapy,
- Available money,

- Available therapeutic resources, and
- Therapist and family time constraints.

Any or all of these issues can profoundly influence the shape and effectiveness of any intervention.

Finally, the question of which therapy or therapies come into play is subject to significant therapist bias (as well as parent bias). In some training centers or geographic locations certain therapies are traditionally recommended and others are considered less valuable, "second best," or unacceptable. For example, individual, intensive, dynamically oriented long-term work may be seen as optimal, with group therapy and pharmacotherapy seen as undesirable "also rans." Pharmacotherapy may be viewed as the treatment of choice with little or no attention given to family work or school consultation. Short-term work may be considered a "treatment failure." Family therapy is sometimes considered the only treatment of choice.

The child psychiatrist in training will do well to question and avoid such doctrinaire positions. Studies comparing the effectiveness of various modalities of treatment are virtually nonexistent. (1) Furthermore, all of these modalities can contribute to progress and combinations of them frequently accelerate the resolution of pathological processes and the facilitation of development. Clinical acumen, flexibility, and open-mindedness are valuable assets for the child psychiatrist as therapist.

Reference

1. McDermott JF (ed): Psychotherapy with children and adolescents (special section). J Am Acad Child Psychiatry 23:527–568, 1984

Chapter 7

Therapeutics I: The Psychotherapies

Kenneth S. Robson, M.D.

In this chapter the major forms of psychotherapeutic intervention will be discussed. These modes should not be rigidly construed as separate therapeutic entities. Rather, many treatment plans involve flexible utilization of parent work, family work, individual child therapy, and group therapy either in their own right or in combination with other forms of intervention.

The psychotherapies involve a central role for the relationship between therapist and patients. The strength of this relationship, and the manner in which it is used, are seen as the agents of change. In fostering change, some or all of the following mechanisms are posited to be significant:

- Support
- Identification with a healthy person
- Provision of a real relationship that replaces a lost or missing one in the child's or family's life, thereby facilitating development
- Insight and reworking of earlier or current psychic trauma
- The learning of new modes of intrapsychic and interper-

sonal relatedness that enhance self-esteem, autonomy, and coping skills
- Time-out: the creation of a calm, soothing, tolerant, and "ego-related" atmosphere within which to heal and grow

Indications for selecting a particular form of psychotherapy are not available at present; there are too little data comparing outcomes. Bias thrives in such a vacuum. Traditionally, intensive individual and parent therapies evolving out of the child guidance movement and psychoanalysis were thought suitable only for better organized children and families with moderate forms of psychopathology. However, at one point in time, intensive psychotherapy with autistic children was also in vogue. Indeed, certain children with autistic features or schizophrenia appear to benefit from individual psychotherapy. With the onset of the community mental health movement, many more poor and disorganized families and their children were referred to child psychiatric programs, and psychotherapies with these populations can be critically important.

However, because the elaboration of criteria for utilization of the psychotherapies requires further study, the child psychiatrist may find the following guidelines helpful:

- All children can benefit from a caring relationship with an adult. Psychotherapy, however, is a scarce, expensive, problem-solving resource. Hence, the nature of the essential problems for child, parents, or family should be clearly identified before referral is made. The need for a friend is not an indication for psychotherapy. Common indications for a child include the following:
  - Treatment of symptoms
  - Enhancement of ego skills (e.g., impulse control, reality testing)
  - Mourning of a loss
  - Resolution of a developmental crisis
  - Clarification of life events (e.g., divorce, sexual abuse)
  - Facilitation of interpersonal skills

- Acceptance of deviance (e.g., mental retardation, birth defects, psychotic parent).

- Most children, regardless of diagnosis, can profit from some forms of psychotherapeutic intervention. The concept of "good patients" is hazardous.
- Families with better organizational skills for scheduling and regular attendance can more easily (although not necessarily more usefully) engage in psychotherapies.
- A child's or family's need for psychotherapy, if difficult to implement initially, should not eliminate subsequent introduction of these modes. For more definitive discussion of psychotherapeutic modes, the reader is referred elsewhere (1–9).
- The beginning therapist may assume that long-term therapies are more desirable or effective than short-term interventions, regardless of therapeutic modality. Such value judgments are not based on comparative outcome data. Experienced therapists know that brief therapeutic experiences often lead to dramatic results. On the other hand, long-term work may be essential. An unbiased position that views the task of any therapy as doing *as little as necessary* to facilitate the child's development can be a helpful guide.

Parent Work

Whatever therapies the treatment plan for a particular child involves, effective intervention with the parents or parent surrogates is *crucial*. No matter how skilled the therapist or how superior the resources, change will not take place without an adequate alliance with the parents. The child who does not have permission to be in therapy can profit little or none from any form of intervention, including hospitalization or residential treatment. Hence, parent work becomes the cornerstone of all therapies.

The child psychiatrist in training is oriented toward patients. It is important to keep in mind that parents do not consciously engage the therapist with concerns of their own;

they are not and should not be treated as patients. One must relate to them as parents, and the tasks are to enhance their empathic skills and help them modulate levels of stimulation around their child—in short, to render them the "facilitating environment." From this perspective it follows that, at least initially, even in the face of gross parental psychopathology, the clinician focuses attention on the child's difficulties and the parent's reactions to them. The alliance is made with the "good parent," that aspect of the parent committed to the child's growth and development. The clinician who has children of his or her own easily appreciates the complexity, frustration, ambivalence, and despair that are normal to the tasks of parenting. One can maintain appropriate professional distance and still empathically share this part of personal life.

The role of the parent therapist should be clear. Worried and insecure parents are often willing to turn over their child to the idealized therapist as "perfect parent." The gratification of such a position for the therapist is seductive but not useful; vigilance is important to avoid this pitfall. The parent therapist's function is to strengthen and enhance existing parent skills, not to erode them further. The useful role is as *facilitator* and *collaborator*, not usurper. The powerful resistance to successful child therapy that conscious or unconscious fears of separation pose to parents have been discussed previously. In this vein it can be useful to remind parents that their job is in some respects like no other: The better they perform, the more they relinquish their parental responsibilities as their child develops toward separation and autonomy.

Another recurrent difficulty for the clinician working with parents is the intense reactions to particular kinds of parental attitudes and behaviors. Psychodynamically, these reactions fall under the rubric of "countertransference." Some of the common parental behaviors that can interfere with the child psychiatrist's alliance include physical or sexual abuse, other forms of sadism, neglect, and overt rejection. Such behaviors generally reflect the parent's own experiences as a child and are a form of "identification with the aggressor." It is the therapist's task to maintain a nonjudgmental, empathic stance. At the same time, anxiety and denial must not stop the therapist from setting appropriate limits that sometimes include legal interventions. Beginning therapists can confuse sadistic and omnipotent impulses of their own with necessary directness and assertiveness essential for the protection of both child and parent.

In addition to these attitudinal considerations of parent therapy, the practical parameters of time, place, and person are important. In traditional psychotherapy the parents are generally seen once weekly by the social workers who work closely with the child's therapist. This team approach can, however, be cumbersome as it requires intense and regular communication, additional time, and money. In private practice, particularly with preadolescent children, one therapist for parents, child, and family is efficient and effective. The primary indications for co-therapy are for children 12 years or older and in clinical situations that require separation of child and parent "boundaries." However, both of these criteria should be used flexibly because they do not apply in many circumstances.

Some practical guidelines for parent therapy include the following:

- With a child in weekly individual therapy, parent meetings should occur *at least* twice monthly and *optimally* weekly as well.
- Brief meetings with parents, 10 to 15 minutes, are sometimes utilized to spare parents a second trip to the clinic/office. This practice is extremely limiting and should be discouraged; alternating weekly sessions with child and parents are more likely to produce therapeutic change.
- Co-therapists should meet or speak by telephone at least twice monthly and should meet together with parents in some regularly scheduled fashion.
- Parents should be encouraged to communicate unexpected and important life events (e.g., illness, loss, death of a pet, school crisis, family disturbance) to the child's therapist *before* he or she sees the child. Communication by phone the night before, a note handed to the therapist, or 2 or 3

minutes in the office before the session begins are usually equally effective.
- Regarding confidentiality, parents should be told that transactions between child and therapist generally remain private. Obviously, in situations of risk or danger to the child, this cannot be the case.

FAMILY WORK

The role of family therapeutic efforts in child therapies varies enormously with training, setting, and clinical circumstances. Furthermore, therapy and models range from family therapy as the exclusive mode to more flexible use of family meetings as they seem clinically indicated. At present, rigid or doctrinaire positions do not seem warranted by the available data on therapeutic outcome. Indications for and contraindications to family approaches are unclear and, in the words of one experienced family therapist, are "if it works." The thoughtful clinician will explore the utility of family work from many perspectives because it is powerful and cost-effective. There is probably no therapeutic plan where some family efforts cannot prove useful. Common situations that may call for family therapeutic experience include:

- Discussion of "family secrets" revealed by a child or parents in individual therapy.
- The need to obtain parental "permission" for a child to speak openly about particular sensitive feelings or events with the therapist.
- Intervention in a family crisis.
- Mourning of a dead, dying, or absent family member.
- Review of custodial arrangements in divorce and separation.
- The failure of individual, group, or other therapeutic modalities.
- Fiscal constraints.

INDIVIDUAL CHILD PSYCHOTHERAPY

Several excellent texts on play therapy with children deal with its history as well as theory and technique. Initial convictions regarding suitability for individual child therapy included sufficient intelligence, moderate levels of disturbance, and ego strengths. Such criteria may loosely speak to health but are unnecessarily restrictive and unsupported by existing studies. Furthermore, because the greater part of therapeutic change generally resides in modifying parental functioning as a facilitating environment, the role of the child's therapy per se as a change agent is uncertain or even obscure.

The concept of "individual" child therapy may also be misstated and, at times, antitherapeutic. In general, the psychotherapist is intervening within a family or child/environment system. The target, so to speak, is the *interface* in these relations between the child and the child's world that contributes to overstimulation, parental empathic failure, and developmental deviance. This latter perception of individual psychotherapy cannot so easily isolate work with the child from the whole therapeutic enterprise. Rather than a sequestered, special, "closed" relationship with the child, even in individual child therapy, the *primary goal* becomes improving the facilitating environment.

Nevertheless, there are many uses to which a working alliance with a child can be put in the service of facilitating development. These include a corrective relationship with a caring, empathic but not overstimulating adult. As noted in Figure 1 (Chapter 6), and within the context of and "held" by the corrective relationship, specific aspects of the child's behavior, perceptions, symptoms, and interpersonal relations can be modified in psychotherapy. For example:

- The modification of maladaptive behavior patterns, personality styles, and character traits.
- Facilitation of movement into a new developmental phase.
- Increased affect tolerance.
- Improved self-esteem.

- Correction of distorted views of reality events and experiences.
- Reduction of inhibition and constriction.
- Strengthened coping skills.
- More effective interpersonal skills.
- Enhanced classroom learning.
- Hopefulness in living.

Obviously, there are many goals that a therapist may wish to pursue in treating a child. The experienced clinician can often work simultaneously on several developmental tasks. But the beginning child therapist should be rigorous in setting therapeutic priorities; that is, what developmental tasks or lines, what problem areas, if addressed, are likely to facilitate developmental progression.

As noted in earlier sections of this manual, the clinical approach to children and child therapy can feel intimidating, anxiety-arousing, and confusing. Sorting out "signal" from "noise" as clinical data emerge can seem impossible. To attempt less, set modest goals, and enjoy one's self with a child are sound starting points. The essential condition for the therapeutic process to prosper is to establish and maintain empathic contact with the child. If the therapist remains aware of the child's emotional state at any point in time, the nature of the therapeutic response becomes self-evident. The content of play and the choice of toys can be seen as clues to the inner affect states and current or past needs of the child. In this way the therapist's choreography and timing mirror those of the empathic parent who senses what is right, how much of it, and when.

The latter point deserves discussion. In one therapeutic session with any child, much may have occurred (the week, night, or hour before) about which the therapist knows little or nothing and will not learn more until later. The child's affect guides the response (e.g., "you seem sad today"). Further, in the course of a session, many shifts of play and behavior will occur. To listen for the affect "driving" these shifts is to disregard distraction and tune in to the simple, central feeling state like the recurrent voice of the French Horn in a symphony—it is enough; all else is elaboration.

In the history of child psychotherapy the importance of fantasy and its meanings was an important contribution of psychoanalysis. However, in the practice of contemporary child psychiatry where weekly, bi-monthly, or less frequent sessions are the rule, the role of fantasy requires reassessment. It is impossible within individual play therapy to sort out reality-based from "imagined" contributions to any play sequence. However, it is generally safer, more accurate, and information-revealing initially to consider all play sequences as reality-based—as portraying some (traumatic?) aspect of the child's external world. Such an orientation both improves the likelihood of appropriate and helpful therapeutic interventions with the child and guides useful sessions to parents who from shame, anxiety, or unawareness will not be aware of some critically important experience in the child's outside world.

Finally, another consideration is the role of games in individual child therapy. Their primary purpose is to establish and maintain "ego-relatedness" (Winnicott) with the child. As such they should be pleasant experiences for both child and therapist. How the child plays (e.g., intensely, regularly breaking rules, always losing) and what games are important data—but data secondary to the need for establishing and maintaining good contact. In this sense process is more important than content.

In conducting individual psychotherapy with children, the beginning therapist, regardless of the choice of responses to the patient, wishes to be liked by the child. This wish is particularly intense in beginning therapists who tend to be rejection-sensitive with their child patients. The child who is aloof, combative, or deliberately hurtful of the therapist's feelings is doing so for some defensive or communicative purpose. Hence, such behaviors should be taken seriously but not too seriously.

GROUP THERAPY

Group psychotherapy in childhood and adolescence is a cost-effective, powerful, and probably underutilized modality of treatment. Troubled interpersonal relationships generally accompany most forms of disturbance in childhood and adolescence. Furthermore, the establishment of good friendships and the strength of group process can rapidly modify intrapsychic problems such as insecurity, low self-esteem, poorly controlled aggression, envy, and difficulty in sharing. Peer pressure appears to be particularly powerful in shaping narcissistic behaviors in children who will relinquish such behaviors often with dramatic speed in a group therapeutic setting. Also, children with special problems (e.g., family dissolution in divorce, serious medical illness, foster care status, mentally ill parents) seem to find ventilation of their concerns more easily in the group context than in individual therapeutic relationships. In adolescence the developmental thrust toward independence may render the group a less intense and regressive environment than one-to-one therapy. Nevertheless, no absolute criteria for selecting individual rather than group therapy in childhood exist and such decisions probably depend on the training of the referring clinician, the availability of a group therapist, and access to adequate space and play materials.

Because peer groups normally begin to form in the early school-age years (7 to 8), therapeutic groups rarely involve children below this age. Thereafter, whether in clinics, schools, or institutional settings, groups of four to eight children run by one or two therapists appear to thrive. With children and early adolescents, play and shared activities are more important therapeutic modes than verbal communication. With mid and late adolescents, of course, talking becomes more useful within the group context. Group psychotherapy should never be seen as a second class service; it has much to offer.

REFERENCES

1. Adams PA: A Primer of Child Psychotherapy, 2nd ed. Boston, Little, Brown and Co, 1982

2. Simmons JE: Psychiatric Examination of Children, 3rd ed. Philadelphia, Lea & Febiger, 1981

3. Group for the Advancement of Psychiatry: The Process of Child Therapy. New York, Brunner/Mazel, 1982

4. Barker P: Basic Child Psychiatry, 4th ed. Baltimore, University Park Press, 1983

5. Connell HM: Essentials of Child Psychiatry. London, Blackwell Scientific Publications, 1979

6. Haworth MR (ed): Child Psychotherapy. New York, Basic Books, 1964

7. McDermott JF, Harrison SI (eds): Psychiatric Treatment of the Child. New York, Jason Aronson, 1977

8. Rutter M, Hersov L: Child Psychiatry: Modern Approaches. London, Blackwell Scientific Publications, 1977

9. Slavson SR, Schiffer M: Group Psychotherapies for Children. New York, International Universities Press, 1975

Chapter 8

Therapeutics II: Intensive Milieu Therapy, Behavior Therapy, and Hypnosis

In this chapter three additional forms of therapeutic intervention will be reviewed. They are grouped together as modalities that can either supplement or, in some instances, provide alternatives to traditional psychotherapies (this is also the case for pharmacotherapy, but because of the size and complexity of the subject, Chapter 9 is devoted exclusively to pharmacotherapy). Intensive milieu therapy encompasses those settings and programs within which the most seriously disturbed children are diagnosed and treated. In many such programs behavior therapy ("behavior modification") is one facilitator of therapeutic change; this approach can and often is utilized as well in outpatient therapeutics. Hypnosis is used sparingly in contemporary child psychiatry and its utility is least clear of all available techniques discussed in this manual. Hypnotic therapies should only be attempted in skilled hands by those who know such techniques and their hazards *as applied to children*; nonetheless, unfamiliarity with this approach should not prevent clinicians from exploring its potential advantages in treating certain conditions, including phobias, "habit disorders," encopresis, enuresis, and the intractable pain of terminal cancers.

Intensive Milieu Therapy for Severely Disturbed Children

Virginia S. Villani, M.D.

The term "severely disturbed" denotes a child's *level of disturbance* rather than a specific diagnosis. Emotional problems of this magnitude are sufficiently extensive to interfere in major ways with family and social relations, school performance, self-esteem, and development itself. The manifestations of disturbance within the families of these children range from complete social isolation to violence toward others. Within the school setting learning is impaired and behaviors that cause disruption of the classroom and school life are the rule. In unstructured social settings the severely disturbed child is an obvious "outsider," unable to relate appropriately to peers. The child's internal world is colored by rejection sensitivity, poorly regulated self-esteem, varying degrees of disorganization of thinking, cognitive delays, and impaired reality-testing. The more common diagnoses in children with severe disturbance are autism, pervasive developmental disorders, schizophrenia and conduct disorders. It is, however, their behaviors, not the diagnoses per se, that bring these children to treatment. More often these behaviors render the child or others unsafe, and include suicidal threats or attempts, firesetting, aggression toward others, premature sexual behavior, and fecal soiling. Some of these behaviors can be managed within the context of family life if the parents are actively engaged in treatment and not contributing unduly to the child's difficulties. On the other hand, even the most well-intentioned, therapeutically oriented parents cannot transform their homes into an intensive treatment milieu for many seriously troubled youngsters.

Referral to an intensive treatment setting most often follows failure in outpatient treatment. The latter may even be bypassed if the presenting symptom is an emergency that precipitates hospitalization. A careful history taken at this time usually reveals ongoing and serious prior symptoms that were unrecognized. Obviously, the need for intensive treatment results when outpatient treatment and regular school services are insufficient either to change the child's behavior or to render the child educable. Hopefully, definitive treatment of the severely disturbed child may prevent the development of disabling adult life psychopathology.

INTENSIVE TREATMENT SETTINGS

Therapeutic settings vary according in their degree of restrictiveness. The child psychiatrist's task is to choose the least restrictive, yet effective, setting. Although hospitalization of the severely disturbed child may be indicated, this alternative is generally time-limited (30, 60, or 90 days) and rarely provides definitive treatment. The indication for hospitalization often centers on questions of safety, diagnostic clarification, or psychopharmacological evaluation. Referral is then made to an appropriate intensive treatment setting. All treatment settings have a therapeutic milieu and most of them use the team approach. Following are the common settings available in this country, arranged from most to least restrictive.

Hospital-Based Treatment Facility

There are very few hospitals that provide long-term psychiatric treatment for children. The few that remain are reserved for the most disturbed children whose medical management or suicidality warrants the kind of supervision that only a hospital can safely provide. These children include, for example, the chronically suicidal or homicidal child, the child with severe self-mutilating behavior, the severe anorectic, and the child with co-existing medical illness and psychological problems whose medical management warrants nursing and physician care.

Residential School

This placement provides the child with 24-hour-a-day year-round services. Many institutions of this kind euphemistically call themselves a "school," although not every residential school is a total care facility. Although children may go home on passes for holidays or weekends, the facility is open at all times. Staffing generally involves child care workers with support staff that include physicians, nurses, social workers, psychologists, teachers, occupational therapists, and recreational therapists. Education is provided on the grounds of the setting. It is important to consider the composition of the staff when choosing a particular residential program. Depending on the diagnosis of the child and the child's medical needs, the availability of trained personnel in specific areas can become a crucial factor in optimal care.

Day Hospital

The psychiatric day hospital provides the same service as a residential school but is located within or closely affiliated with a medical facility. Children are sent home at the end of the day and on weekends and holidays. The program day itself is usually longer than the average school day in order to provide after-school therapeutic groups. Such a program requires a high degree of family involvement, particularly around safety issues and therapeutic management of the child. As an alternative to residential treatment, day hospitals can treat severely disturbed children while allowing them to live with their families of origin or suitable foster care. Thus more long-term intensive family work and less environmental disruption become possible.

Group Homes

Group homes provide residence for children who cannot live at home either for behavioral or emotional reasons. The group home model operates from the premise that family life may not be tolerable for some disturbed children. Such children have usually suffered severe emotional trauma within the context of a family such that intimacy becomes fraught with conflict. Some have experienced multiple unsuccessful foster care placements. With group homes children may spend weekends and holidays either in their own homes or in that of an extended family or foster family. Educational services may be provided on the grounds of the group home or within the local public school system.

Therapeutic Day School

A day school program is a private school for the education of the severely disturbed child. Many schools have an affiliation with an outpatient clinic that may provide both individual therapy for the children and family work. Rarely does a school provide all services. The emphasis of the therapeutic day school is clearly educational since after-school and summer programs are not routinely provided.

PRACTICAL ASPECTS OF PLACEMENT CHOICE

Once the determination that a child needs a comprehensive treatment approach is made, the clinician is faced with the complex task of actually obtaining it. This is a joint venture between parents or guardian and clinicians, with the clinician taking a firm, guiding stance. Placement of such a child is seriously hindered by dwindling state and local financial resources. All the settings described above are expensive and most private insurance carriers do not cover such services. These are private facilities, supported by wealthy families who can afford to send their children. For the most part, however, treatment facilities are funded through public monies from the social service agencies or the public school system, or through a cost-shared approach from both. Public law 94-142, which mandates all local public schools to provide an education for every child from ages 3 to 21, regardless of emotional or physical handicaps, has different methods of implementation in every state (1). For clinical purposes it is critical to be familiar with the local administration of this act. Similarly, the availability of public monies through social services, mental health agencies, or juvenile service agencies is closely tied to local politics and traditions. It behooves the skilled child psychiatrist to become thoroughly acquainted with these fiscal and political issues as they directly impact ability to advocate successfully for the needs of the child.

The process of finding the best placement for the child often requires months. However, the need should be anticipated as early as possible, which may mean beginning to plan for a child's next school year in March, or raising the question of an out-of-home setting early in the course of a psychiatric inpatient evaluation. For the most part, there is a dearth of facilities and an abundance of children in need. Given the expense, and the need for public monies, bureaucratic entanglements are common. Many states have child advocacy agencies that can be helpful in the placement process. Exploring available openings in local facilities is an essential task for the clinician and parents or guardian. The following issues should be addressed in investigating particular settings:

- What particular kind of child does the facility treat?
- What is the program's treatment orientation?
- How long has the program been in existence?
- How are families involved?
- What is the professional composition of the staff?
- What is a typical day in the life of the child like?
- What happens on weekends and holidays?
- How is the program funded and is this funding stable?

Once appropriate settings have been identified, visiting them for preadmission interviews and touring *always* is indicated. During the entire process, close collaboration among clinician, parents or guardian, and funding source is critical. The role of the child psychiatrist as clinician should be to help coordinate efforts in the best interests of the child. It is also important to keep the child well-informed that everyone is working together in his or her behalf. When appropriate, the child should be actively involved in the planning and its progress. In summary, the arduous task of obtaining proper treatment for the severely disturbed child requires the skilled clinician to have a thorough understanding of child psychopathology as well as local political and social realities. The integration of this knowledge for the child's benefit is crucial if effective treatment is to be obtained.

SOME BASIC PRINCIPLES IN TREATING THE SEVERELY DISTURBED CHILD

Because the child's disturbance reaches into every area of the child's life, the treatment must be both extensive and lengthy. In most instances this involves long-term treatment of at least 1 year, and often several years. An integration of all therapeutic approaches applicable to the child's daily life routine is essential. Most therapeutic settings utilize a combination of individual treatment, family therapy or family work, group therapy, behavior modification, and pharmacotherapy. The relative balance between these approaches depends on the orientation and training of the service setting. All of these modalities combine to form the "therapeutic milieu," a term that denotes the environment that surrounds the child. The milieu is an essential aspect of the treatment and has received much attention by Bettelheim and Sanders (2), Aichorn (3), and Redl (4), among others. These authors contribute to an understanding of the vicissitudes and rewards of treating the severely disturbed child.

The effectiveness of treatment depends on an integration of the child within groups while simultaneously individualizing treatment. Further, treatment modalities become adapted to the specific developmental stage of the child. For example, a comprehensive plan requires an appreciation of normal developmental stages, detailed knowledge of the child's psychopathology, a thorough understanding of the treatment modalities available, and knowledge of how children function in groups, with attention to how the child in question will function with peers in a particular setting.

Given these complexities, a treatment team approach is essential. The team consists of representatives from various parts of the program and is, therefore, multidisciplinary in nature. It is usually composed of the child's therapist, an educational staff member (often the teacher), a child care worker, a medical person (nurse or psychiatrist), and the child's family worker. The team must meet frequently to review goals, communicate new data, and adjust treatment plans. The optimal role of the child psychiatrist as the most comprehensively trained clinician and often, as well, the child's therapist is to *lead* the team. Such leadership must be done in a tactful and facilitating manner that allows for maximal participation. If the child psychiatrist is to assume this role, he or she must be closely involved with the milieu, a task that requires substantial time and effort outside of the therapeutic time. The risk of psychotherapy becoming split from the milieu is a common pitfall. Within the private sector/nonacademic settings, the team leader role is more variable and may be assumed by the child's therapist, who is often not a physician or a consultant. The leader's task, however, is to integrate all staff members' work with the child around *agreed on*, specific goals.

The primary goals of treatment of the severely disturbed child are *to facilitate development* and *to render the child able to function in a less restrictive setting*. Such "healthier" functioning, however, must be integrated into the child's psyche. If it is merely obtained through "training" of the child, the child will be unable to sustain the "cure" once outside of the treatment setting, and symptoms will reemerge. This variable, the durability of the long-term treatment outcome, is still an area of controversy and confusion. Doctrinaire positions are to be avoided.

Behavior Therapy

Janet Gillmore, Ph.D.

Behavior therapy is an alternative or complementary method of treatment within the field of child psychiatry. Its utility for psychological problems is wide ranging but not all-encompassing (5, 6). The decision to focus on behavior rather than emotions and dynamic issues in a treatment plan depends on careful clinical evaluation in addition to experience and target symptoms that yield to such intervention. Practical concerns over the ability to institute a behavioral program must also be considered. The clinician needs to be in a position of sufficient control, and family members involved must be able to cooperate for a program to succeed. However, when behavior therapy is the treatment of choice and is well executed, it can provide concrete, direct, rapid, and often definitive relief for psychological problems. In general, behavioral approaches should be considered an aspect of the overall treatment plan for any child; traditional therapeutic approaches and behavioral strategies can and do fit together in thoughtful clinical hands.

The first task is to define the goal of a behavioral approach; what is the child to learn and relearn. This task necessitates deriving specific goals from general treatment objectives and subsequently operationalizing the goals into observable, carefully defined behaviors. It is important to select a behavioral goal that is meaningful for treatment (e.g., increased food intake in anorexia nervosa, control in encopresis). However, it is difficult to facilitate change by focusing directly on the most salient and problematic behavior or symptoms. Corollary and contributory behaviors are often the best initial targets.

At the present time, those clinical problems encountered in clinical child psychiatry that appear to be sensitive to behavioral approaches include encopresis, some forms of enuresis, eating patterns in anorexia nervosa, habit disturbances (e.g., trichtillomania, or hair-pulling), and self-mutilating—a disruptive behavior most often seen in populations of institutionalized mentally retarded children. Whatever the target symptom, however, the best outcome from behavior interventions occurs in the context of a comprehensive and unbiased overall psychiatric plan.

Understanding the nature and extent of the clinical problem is a critical step in any treatment formulation. For example, behavior therapy aimed at fecal soiling in a child who is psychotic is likely to fail unless the primary clinical problem is first addressed. From a behavioral perspective, the information-gathering step is essential and provides the foundation for measuring the developing treatment approaches. The emphasis is on systemically and accurately collecting data on the behaviors of concern. First, a clear, specific, and communicable description of the *target behavior* is needed. To obtain reliable data, independent observations must be consistent. An effort must be made to reduce observer bias (i.e., seeing what one expects to see). Also, the same type of observation should be made as both a pre- and postmeasure of the treatment effect. There are a variety of observational techniques and sampling procedures developed that are designed to ensure accurate information collection. Next, the *baseline data* should be gathered for the purpose of assessing the extent of the problem as a starting point for measuring treatment progress. This step should be taken before any intervention is suggested. The clinician needs to select a data collector who can function as an independent, dependable, and unbiased assessor. It usually makes the most sense to select an individual presently in the child's environment (e.g., school personnel, family member).

With the information accumulated, the next phase is to

negotiate a program with all of the parties involved. Reinforcers need to be selected based on the child's interests, needs, and developmental level. The clinician typically conceives of a hierarchy of reinforcers from primary (e.g., food) to social behavior. The appropriate reinforcer will function either to increase or decrease a target behavior. If the child is learning a new or deficient behavior, the reinforcer will help to support the development of it. If there is an excessive behavior, then the reinforcer will function to diminish that response, possibly by having the present reinforcer withdrawn. Also, responses that are incompatible with the maladaptive response can be strengthened. In crediting and negotiating the program, the clinician needs to try to predict the patterns of response. The degree of the patient's cooperation, the length of time, the support of significant others, and the patterns of increasing versus decreasing responsiveness should all be anticipated.

The *schedule* for the program and its contingencies should then be carefully delineated. It is helpful to write down the program, either in chart form or as a contractual agreement. Such a tangible presentation helps to legitimize and validate the program and its importance. A simple, concise format should be clearly understandable to all parties involved. The program agreement should incorporate the time period and dates involved, the goal (the behavior to be charged), the specific reinforcers and their amounts, and the schedule for renegotiating the agreement.

Finally, the treatment plan should be *renegotiated* after a fixed period of time. The specific behavioral goals are further elaborated and structured by the clinician in order to achieve the primary clinical goal. Also, programs need to be adjusted according to problems that arise. Thus the clinician functions as a troubleshooter in the renegotiations. Often the observable changes brought about via a behavioral approach facilitate or ready a child and the child's family for other forms of psychotherapy.

Hypnosis with Children

Joae G. Brooks, M.D.

Hypnosis, like behavior therapies, can be an adjunct to or, occasionally, a primary therapeutic tool with children with certain psychiatric disorders. It has been successfully used—but should by no means be considered the treatment of choice—for anxiety, enuresis, soiling, urinary retention, mutism, functional megacolon, hair pulling, nail biting, obsessive-compulsive symptoms, phobias, school refusal, eczema, asthma, vomiting, psychogenic pain; pain from physical causes, migraine headaches, conversion reactions, learning disability; and the management of anxiety and pain in young burn and cancer patients, in children undergoing minor surgical and dental procedures, and in adolescent girls about to have their first pelvic examination (7–14).

Hypnosis can increase compliance and cooperation, decrease fear, and at the same time provide the child with a feeling of mastery and control. Children are more easily hypnotized because they are more imaginative and able to fantasize than adults; they also possess more cognitive fluidity.

Hypnosis is an altered state of consciousness where the mind's focus is narrowed to certain specific stimuli. Thus what the therapist suggests to the child during a hypnotic trance has greater influence. Initially the child should be given some kind of choice concerning what is about to happen. The child may choose which member of the family is to be present when the procedure is going to be done. If there is a favorite stuffed animal, the child can be asked if the animal should go through the procedure first or if he or she would like to do it on the animal after undergoing the procedure. Being permitted to make a decision makes the child feel that his or her wishes and feelings are important and that the child has at least some control over the situation. Children are eager to hear and take hold of ideas that they think will alleviate their pain and fear.

Andolseek (9) outlines the steps in hypnosis with children and emphasizes the importance of training in these techniques. The first step is to secure the understanding and cooperation of the parents and professionals involved. A trance may be induced by eye fixation on some object (e.g., the therapist's thumb), arm levitation, or progressive muscular relaxation. The therapist must be confident and reassuring. An image of going down a ladder or staircase with muscles becoming heavier and more relaxed with each step is helpful. The child is asked to talk about a recent happy event or holiday or favorite television program in all its sensory-evoking detail, which distracts from the surroundings and narrows and focuses the child's attention. The therapist shows most interest in the child's tale and asks about feelings, colors, sounds, and smells in a positive vein. Part of the environment can be incorporated into the hypnotic induction; Andolseek likens an operating room lamp to the sun and speaks to the child of the warmth of the sun and being at the beach playing. The child is asked to talk about a game he or she likes to play in the sun and in this way the trance can be maintained.

Infants and very young children can be helped by hypnotic techniques. Anxiety in a small child can be reduced by asking the child to carry out a simple, repetitive task like putting pegs into holes or lining up blocks or toy animals. Moore (10) illustrates how, for example, a tense, frightened boy can be helped by being told that he can control how he feels. The child is taught by suggestion to relax, told that he feels good now, and told that he can learn how to have this good feeling whenever he wants. Posthypnotic suggestions can maintain clinical improvement. It is often necessary to conduct several sessions that can be spaced every 2 or 3 days or weekly to eradicate symptoms and increase the child's confidence in this new way of having control.

Gardner (14) states that hynosis is not likely to be helpful if the child is not motivated to change the habit. The child may derive too much pleasure or secondary gain to want to give it up. Gardner feels that hypnosis should not be used for symptom removal if the symptom binds severe anxiety or wards off depression. In such instances psychotherapy must precede any use of hypnosis. Gardner has not observed symptom substitution following the proper use of hynotherapy in children. The appropriate role of hypnosis in child psychiatry remains to be determined.

REFERENCES

1. Palfrey JS: Commentary on PL 94-142: The Education for All Handicapped Children Act. J Pediatr 97:417–419, 1980

2. Bettelheim B, Sanders J: Milieu therapy: the orthogenic school model, in Basic Handbook of Child Psychiatry, Vol III: Therapeutic Interventions. Edited by Noshpitz JD, Harrison SI. New York, Basic Books, 1979

3. Aichorn A: Wayward Youth. New York, Viking Press, 1939

4. Redl F: Children Who Hate. Glencoe, Ill, Free Press, 1951

5. Wolpe J: The Practice of Behavior Therapy. New York, Pergamon Press, 1969

6. Graziano A, Mooney K: Children and Behavior Therapy. Chicago, Aldine, 1984

7. Gardner GG: Hypnotherapy in management of childhood habit disorders. J Pediatr 92:835–840, 1978

8. Olness K: Hypnosis in pediatric practice. Curr Probl Pediatr 12:1–47, 1981

9. Andolseek K: Use of hypnosis with children. J Fam Pract 10:503–507, 1980

10. Moore CL: Hypnosis: an adjunct to pediatric consultation. Am J Clin Hypn 23:211–216, 1981

11. Podoll E: The use and misuse of hypnosis in children. Journal of the American Society of Psychosomatic Dentistry and Medicine 28:57–59, 1981

12. Elkins GR, Carter BD: Use of a science-fiction-based imagery technique in child hypnosis. Am J Clin Hypn 23:274–277, 1981

13. Williams DT, Singh M: Hypnosis as a facilitating therapeutic adjunct in child psychiatry. J Am Acad Child Psychiatry 15:326–342, 1976

14. Gardner GG: Hypnosis with infants and preschool children. Am J Clin Hypn 19:158–162, 1977

Chapter 9

Therapeutics III: Pharmacotherapy

Barbara J. Coffey, M.D.

GENERAL APPROACHES TO DRUG THERAPY

Psychopharmacologic agents have been used to treat childhood disturbances for many years, but only recently has the era of modern scientific pediatric psychopharmacology begun.

The present-day child psychiatrist or pediatrician can choose from all of the categories of psychotropic agents available to the general psychiatrist or adult practitioner. Knowledge of the basic principles of psychotropic drug use, the work-up for use of these drugs in childhood, the basic categories of drugs, their indications, and side effect profiles is crucial for the up-to-date child clinician. This knowledge can then be competently applied to the practical use of these agents in the clinical setting in childhood and adolescence.

Indications

Despite recent advances in research strategies and methodology in pediatric psychopharmacology, there are still few formal indications for psychoactive drug use in childhood and adolescence. Drugs, like all forms of therapy in child psychiatry, are to be used to promote optimal development and maturation, or to assist in the removal of obstacles for development to proceed onward in an adaptive fashion. In most cases, drug therapy represents one component of a total treatment plan for the child, including other forms of therapy. Quite frequently, medication can be used to help make the disturbed child more responsive to other forms of therapy.

Established indications will be discussed in the section that follows on specific agents. General indications for drug therapy include the following categories of disturbance:

- Childhood and adolescent psychosis
- Severe behavioral disturbance accompanying mental retardation or child psychiatric emergencies
- Tourette's syndrome
- Enuresis
- Attention deficit disorder with hyperactivity
- Some forms of sleep disturbance

Other conditions in which indications are informally established at present but are potentially drug responsive include:

- Childhood depression
- Separation anxiety disorder
- Anxiety states
- Borderline states
- Sleep arousal disorders

General Guidelines to Drug Therapy in Childhood and Adolescence

Frequently children and adolescents are not self-referred for psychiatric intervention; often they are not even willing patients. In most cases, the child's behavior or emotional state is disturbing to someone else in the environment, usually an adult such as a parent or teacher. The *parent's attitude* toward the use of medication and ability to work with the doctor and child is extremely important. A parent is a necessary source of information about the child's functioning and response to medication. The parent and often the teacher need to be informed about the reasons for the drug therapy, the likely therapeutic effects, side effects, and toxicities. A child with an unreliable parent who cannot observe, administer, and monitor the medication may not be treatable with pharmacotherapy. As there are few formal diagnostic indications for pharmacotherapy in childhood, and diagnostic criteria themselves such as the *Diagnostic and Statistical Manual of Mental Disorders, Third Edition (DSM-III)* (1) have some limitations in applicability in child psychiatry, it is useful to approach drug therapy on a *problem-oriented* or *target-symptom* basis. The clinician should, in a cohesive and relevant way, draw up a list of problems or target symptoms with which the child presents. Common target symptoms that are potentially drug responsive include attentional difficulties, hyperactivity, enuresis, tics, and sleep disturbance such as insomnia or night terrors. Although establishing a diagnosis is important for each child, it is frequently the target symptom that will guide the clinician as to choice of agent.

Children differ significantly from adults in their *pharmacokinetic* capacities. Children have relatively large liver size in proportion to body weight when compared with adults and after about a year of age reach adult glomerular filtration rates; therefore they seem to function metabolically more efficiently with regard to drug handling. Often children tend to need higher doses relative to body weight when compared to adults (2).

In addition, evidence suggests that children tend to have less adipose tissue and less protein binding, when compared to adults, and may have more drug available for bioactivity and, potentially, side effects (3).

Growth and development itself are associated with changes in organ size and proportion and in tissue mass, particularly water and adipose tissue. These changes may have significant effects on drug handling. Adolescents approach adults in their metabolic and pharmacokinetic parameters.

Appropriate drug selection requires comprehensive information about the child and the child's history, current functioning, family history, and medical history. As the criteria for drug selection with this patient population are not always clearly defined, it behooves the clinician to try to select the most likely to be effective and least toxic agent that is available. The clinician should be knowledgeable about and have familiarity with one or two agents and their dosage ranges and side effect profiles in each category.

Dosage regulation requires time and experience. Few guidelines are available in the literature (4). In general, calculating initial dose and ceiling dose on a milligrams per kilogram basis is useful, particularly with the antidepressants and psychostimulants. Plasma levels of some drugs can be readily obtained, and therapeutic ranges similar to those of adults have been identified, such as with the tricyclic antidepressants and lithium carbonate. In general, except in emergencies, it is best to start with a low dosage and raise by standardized increments every 2 or 3 days until therapeutic effects or range is reached or until the onset of side effects. Often it is necessary to push the dosage up to the point of development of side effects in order to explore the optimal range. Frequently the dosage can then be gradually lowered to find a balance between minimum necessary for therapeutic effect and minimal possibility of side effects.

In the case of the acutely psychotic child with target symptoms of motor overactivity, delusional thinking or hallucinations, and agitation, or the acutely assaultive child in an emergency state, medication can be given more frequently until the child is sedated or calmed. In this situation oral (p.o.) concentrates can be given every 1 or 2 hours until a therapeutic effect is achieved.

Side effects are not infrequent in childhood and adolescence, although they may be transient or of little clinical significance. Many of the side effects of neuroleptic, antidepressant medication and lithium seen in adult patients can be seen in children and adolescents. Of particular concern are the anticholinergic and cardiovascular side effects of the tricyclic antidepressants and the extrapyramidal side effects of the neuroleptics, including dyskinesias (5, 6). Withdrawal dyskinesias seem to be more frequent than tardive dyskinesia (TD) in young children, but TD has been observed in this age group.

Duration of treatment will depend upon the target symptom, the age of the child, the kind of psychotropic agent, and the unique features of the clinical situation. There are few fixed guidelines as to length of time on the medications, drug holiday programs, and indications for stopping. In general, if a child has not responded to an agent within 4 weeks while in the therapeutic range, it is unlikely he or she will respond at a later date. A rational approach to this situation would be to switch to another drug in the same category or to another category altogether if indicated.

Most children with a therapeutic response to medication will need a 3- to 6-month trial of the agent, depending on the clinical situation. Some will require a longer period of time. In general, no child or adolescent should remain on any agent for more than a year without at least a 1- to 2-month drug holiday.

Periodic drug holidays are indicated for all psychotropic agents for two reasons: (a) to reassess the child's need for the agent at regular intervals and (b) to monitor for the development of side effects such as growth changes or dyskinesias.

THE BASIC WORK-UP

The Predrug Work-up

All child and adolescent patients who are candidates for psychopharmacologic agents should undergo a thorough medical and psychiatric evaluation. The clinical work-up should include a *comprehensive psychiatric evaluation*, including:

- Chief complaint(s) and target symptoms.
- Present illness.
- Past psychiatric history and treatment(s).
- Family history including three-generation genogram; medical and/or psychiatric illness, alcoholism, causes of death, and ages at death should be noted. A medication history

for family members with psychiatric illness should be obtained, with responses to medication noted.
- Developmental history, school history, and social history.
- Complete medical history of the child including illnesses, hospitalizations and/or surgery, and allergies.
- Medication history for the child and previous response to medications.
- Mental status examination (see Chapter 2).
- Auxiliary data such as psychometric testing, particularly projectives. These can be helpful in decision making as to class of medication if the child has a constellation of target symptoms that can potentially be treated with more than one type of agent. For example, a child with attentional difficulties and hyperactivity with much depressive affect on projective testing should probably be tried on imipramine hydrochloride first, rather than a stimulant.
- Formulation, working diagnosis, and differential diagnosis.

In addition to a comprehensive psychiatric evaluation, a *complete physical examination* prior to starting medication is of paramount importance. First, for differential diagnostic purposes, physical assessment is necessary to rule out organic sources of the child's disturbance such as temporal lobe seizures or hyperthyroidism. Secondly, all of the agents can have physical effects on the child such as alterations in blood pressure, pulse, or weight. Height, weight, blood pressure, temperature, pulse, and respiration should be noted.

A screening *neurological examination* should be performed on all patients who are candidates for psychotropic agents, noting overall developmental level, gross and fine motor coordination, cranial nerve functions, muscle tone and strength, reflexes, sensory functions, and gait. Before medication is started, note should be made as to the presence or absence of unusual movements, tics, or stereotypic behaviors. These are commonly seen in psychotic youngsters and need to be distinguished from medication-related dyskinesias. (7).

Children with special problems such as heart conditions or seizure disorders may need consultation with a specialist prior to drug therapy.

A *minimal laboratory work-up* for all children who are candidates for medication includes the following:

- Complete blood count (CBC) and differential blood count
- Urinalysis
- Blood urea nitrogen (BUN), creatinine, electrolytes
- Height, weight, and growth chart
- Pregnancy test where appropriate, in sexually active female adolescents
- Toxic screen where appropriate, in substance users
- Lead blood level in the child who presents with hyperactivity

For children who are candidates for *tricyclic antidepressants*, the following are useful baseline parameters:

- Thyroid function tests: T_3, T_4, T_4I, thyroid-stimulating hormone (TSH)
- SMA12 including liver function tests (LFT): protein, albumin, bilirubin (direct and indirect), alkaline phosphatase, serum glutamic oxaloacetic transamine (SGOT), serum glutamic pyruvic transaminase (SGPT), lactic dehydrogenase (LDH), creatine phosphokinase (CPK)
- Electrocardiogram (EKG)
- Electroencephalogram (EEG) may be useful, and necessary in the child with preexisting seizure disorder

For children who are candidates for *neuroleptics* (antipsychotics):

- Add SMA12 including LFTs
- Abnormal Involuntary Movement Screen (AIMS) (8)
- Blood pressure and pulse

For children who are candidates for *psychostimulants*:

- Add Conners checklist (9) for attention deficit disorder with hyperactivity before and it can be repeated after medication. Both parents and teacher can fill out the checklist for

5 to 7 days prior to drug therapy for baseline, then after the child has reached therapeutic range. This can be useful quantitative data in determining drug response.
- Add blood pressure, pulse, height, weight, and growth chart (10).

For children who are candidates for *lithium carbonate*:

- Add SMA12 including LFTs and calcium
- Thyroid function tests as for tricyclics
- Creatinine clearance can be helpful, but not mandatory, if urinalysis, BUN, and creatinine have been obtained

Specialized tests studied in adult psychiatry, such as the dexamethasone suppression test, urinary catecholamines, sleep architecture studies, and hypothalamic-pituitary stimulation tests, have not been clarified for routine clinical use in this age group despite some evidence that they may have some value as research tools.

Written and informed consent of the parent(s) or legal guardian and "assent" of the child may be useful in some cases in which the indications for drug therapy are not formally established, such as use of tricyclic antidepressants for children under 12 with major depression or separation anxiety disorder. But, in general, informed consent is a process that takes place in an ongoing dialogue between doctor and parent(s) and child. The parent and child have the right to know expected therapeutic and adverse effects and relative risks versus benefits. Discussion of these issues in a straightforward, simple fashion can facilitate ongoing communication in most cases.

Careful record-keeping is a must. Note in the record should be made of

- Target symptoms that are being treated with medication.
- Rationale for drug selection.
- Initial dosage and medication plan.
- Increases of dosage and response.
- Presence of any adverse reactions including expected side

effects or any unexpected allergic or idiosyncratic reactions.
- Documentation of discussion with parent(s) and child regarding informed consent issues.
- Rationale for changing or discontinuing drug(s).

Drug Maintenance and Monitoring

Children and adolescents usually need to be seen at regular and frequent intervals during the initiation of drug therapy, at least once a week. Close communication is necessary with the parent during this time as well. Parents should be encouraged to call the doctor if any questions arise about medication. Good communication between doctor and family facilitates beneficial response.

Once the child has been stabilized, usually after several weeks, on a maintenance dosage, a drug maintenance program can begin. Children can generally be seen less frequently, such as monthly, to review therapeutic response and development of side effects. Information from teachers and other clinicians involved in the child's care must be regularly communicated to the prescribing physician.

All children on all pharmacotherapy should have at least one yearly drug holiday to reassess need for the drug and to monitor for the development of side effects. The duration and timing of the drug-free period will vary with the individual child, type of drug, and clinical situation.

Periodic laboratory screening should be done on a regular basis during the entire duration of drug therapy. It is judicious practice to repeat CBC and differential, urinalysis, and basic chemistry screening at 3 months and every 6 months for each of the medications. Certain specific procedures such as EKG monitoring will be discussed in the sections on specific agents (below).

In general, it is very useful to record weight and height on a monthly or quarterly basis, as many of these agents can cause weight gain, or in some cases, weight loss. Keeping the National Center for Health Statistics growth chart (10) can provide the clinician easy access to growth parameters over an extended period of time.

Specific Agents

Neuroleptic (Antipsychotic) Drugs

Neuroleptic medications include the phenothiazines, butyrophenones, thioxanthenes, dibenzoxazepines, and dihydroindolones.

Formal indications for use of these drugs include target symptoms of (a) childhood and adolescent psychoses and pervasive developmental disorders such as agitation, stereotypies, and social withdrawal; (b) severe behavior disturbance as accompaniment to mental retardation such as self-destructive or assaultive behavior; (c) psychiatric emergencies, including acute homicidal behavior and severe disorganizing anxiety/agitation; and (d) Tourette's syndrome.

These medications function as dopamine, α adrenergic, and cholinergic blockers in the central nervous system (CNS) and peripheral nervous system (PNS). They have antipsychotic actions in adults and in children with such target symptoms as auditory hallucinations or delusions. In addition these drugs can decrease severe agitation and motor overactivity, as well as stereotypic movements and postures, and render an apathetic, socially nonrelated psychotic child more amenable to his or her environment (11).

In general, neuroleptics tend to be chosen on their side effect profile rather than on clinical effects, which are approximately equal with comparable doses. The low potency aliphatic and piperidine phenothiazines such as chlorpromazine and thioridazine, respectively, tend to be sedating and more anticholinergic, whereas the high potency butyrophenones and piperazine phenothiazines such as haloperidol and trifluoperazine tend to be less sedating, but more likely to induce extrapyramidal side effects (EPS) such as akathisia, acute dystonic reactions, and parkinsonism. The thioxanthenes and newer dibenzoxazepines and dihydroindolones tend to be intermediate for anticholinergic and EPS (Table 1A).

An agitated child with stereotypic behaviors will generally respond more successfully to a sedating neuroleptic, whereas

Table 1A. Neuroleptics (Antipsychotics) for Use in Children Over 6 Years of Age

Generic Name (Trade Name)	Indications	Oral Dosage Range (mg)	Common Side Effects Short-Term	Common Side Effects Long-Term
Phenothiazines	Pervasive developmental disorders and psychoses, acute or chronic; severe behavioral problems associated with mental retardation; psychiatric emergencies; acute agitation		Autonomic Nervous System: sedation, dry mouth, orthostatic hypotension, urinary retention, blurring of vision	
Chlorpromazine (Thorazine)[a]		10–300		
Thioridazine (Mellaril)[a]		10–300		
Trifluoperazine (Stelazine)[b]		1–20		
Fluphenazine (Prolixin)[b]		1–10		
Perphenazine (Trilafon)[b]		2–24		
Butyrophenones	Tourette's syndrome (Haldol in particular is useful)		*EPS*: acute dystonic reaction, akathisia, Parkinsonism	
Haloperidol (Haldol)[a]		1–16		
Thioxanthenes				Withdrawal and TD
Thiothixene (Navane)[b]		2–20		
Dibenzoxazepines			Endocrine: prolactin, menstrual irregularities	
Loxapine (Loxitane)[c]		5–60		
Dihydroindolones			Hypersensitivity: rash, blood dyscrasias, elevated liver functions	Weight gain
Molindone (Moban)[b]		10–50		
			CNS: seizures, behavioral reactions	

[a]FDA approved for advertising for use in children under 6 years old.
[b]FDA approved for advertising for use in children over 12 years old.
[c]FDA approved for advertising for use in children over 16 years old.

Table 1B. Recommended Neuroleptic (Antipsychotic) Treatment

Suggested Treatment Regimens for Psychosis and Pervasive Developmental Disorders

Chlorpromazine (p.o. tablets or concentrate)
- Start with 0.5–1.0 mg/kg
- Acutely: give 0.5–2.0 mg/kg q 2–4 hours until therapeutic response or side effects; usually 3 or 4 doses will have therapeutic effect
- Daily maintenance dose range: 3–10 mg/kg

Haloperidol (p.o. tablets or concentrate)
- Start with 0.5 mg
- Acutely: give 0.01–0.10 mg/kg q 2–4 hours until therapeutic response or side effects; usually 3 or 4 doses will have therapeutic effect
- Daily maintenance dose range: 0.1–0.5 mg/kg

Suggested Treatment Regimen for Agitation/Anxiety, Psychiatric Emergencies (Aggressive Behavior)
Follow the acute recommendations as above, then discontinue medication as soon as feasible. In some cases hydroxyzine can be used.

Suggested Treatment Regimen for Tourette's Syndrome
Haloperidol
- Start with 0.25 mg for 3–4 days, then increase by 0.25 mg every 5–7 days
- Daily maintenance dose is usually 1.5–10 mg daily

an anergic, withdrawn child should probably be treated with a less sedating drug. Sedation effects must be monitored because an oversedated child cannot learn.

Children and adolescents are like their adult counterparts in that they are at risk for development of autonomic nervous system side effects and EPS.

There is growing evidence that adolescents and even young children can develop neuroleptic-related dyskinesias. Some studies (12) have indicated that children are more likely to develop withdrawal emergent dyskinesias that are reversible on discontinuation of the medication than TD or late-appearing dyskinesias; nevertheless, TD has been reported in young children as well as in adolescents (13). Abnormal movements often present in these disturbed children *prior to* drug treatment must be differentiated from any that develop *after* drug treatment.

In general it is good practice to prescribe the *lowest possible* effective dose for maintenance, and to take the child off the neuroleptic at least once yearly in the case of a chronic psychosis or severe behavioral disturbance associated with mental illness. In the case of a psychiatric emergency such as acute agitation or assaultive behavior, the child should be taken off medication as quickly as possible following return of psychic, family, and environmental equilibrium.

Psychostimulants

The psychostimulants are some of the most widely prescribed and better-studied psychotropic agents in child psychiatry and pediatrics. Methylphenidate, dextroamphetamine, and magnesium pemoline are the agents available for use in this country.

These drugs function as general nonspecific stimulators of catecholamine activity in the CNS and PNS; they appear to prevent catecholamine reuptake at the synaptic cleft as well as inhibit metabolism and breakdown (14). They are formally indicated in the treatment of attention deficit disorder with hyperactivity (minimal brain dysfunction, hyperkinesis in past) and help these children to focus their attention more clearly, slow down their motor activity, and become less distractible. They have had informal use with some conduct disorders and attention deficit disorder without hyperactivity. Their effect actually does not appear to be paradoxical (15) in that adult males and normal boys also appear to increase concentration and focusing when given a single dose of dextroamphetamine. Stimulants appear to achieve their effects by short-term improvement of attentional difficulties and concentration; they have not been shown to have any long-term effects by themselves on achievement or cognition.

Because dextroamphetamine and methylphenidate have a relatively short duration of action with peak effects between 1 and 3 hours, they must be administered in divided doses twice a day or so (16). They are typically given at breakfast and at noontime (or early afternoon). As this may necessitate the child receiving the medication in school, it may sometimes be easier to give it to the child immediately after school as long as it does not interfere with sleep. This may save the child some embarrassment in school from having to go to the school nurse's office everyday. Pemoline, with a longer duration of action and said to have less side effects, can be given once a day before school. There are also slow release forms available for dextroamphetamine and methylphenidate.

One study indicates a differential effect of dosage of methylphenidate on cognitive performance and behavioral symptomatology, with cognitive performance optimal at lower dosages (0.3 mg/kg) than behavior (1.0 mg/kg) (17).

Common side effects include nausea, abdominal discomfort, anorexia, and insomnia. There have been some reports of adverse effects on growth parameters that are reversible with discontinuation of the medication (18, 19), but other evidence has been contradictory. A potentially serious side effect is the development of Tourette's syndrome in the vulnerable child, so that a preexisting tic or family history of tics is in most cases a contraindication for use. Stimulants may precipitate psychotic symptomatology including hallucinosis in children at risk. Methylphenidate seems to be less likely to produce side effects than dextroamphetamine.

All drugs in this group should generally be given on a drug-holiday basis to mitigate the potential for side effects. Weekends, school vacations, summer vacations, and the first month of school in the fall should be drug-free periods.

Antidepressants

The use of tricyclic antidepressants in child psychiatry has grown in the past few years; they now appear to have widespread use in several conditions, although still largely informal.

The tricyclic antidepressants are formally established for use in children with enuresis and hyperactivity/attention deficit disorders. In addition, tricyclic antidepressants have been studied for use in conduct disorders, childhood depression, and school refusal based on separation anxiety (3). Tricyclic antidepressants have also been used in sleep arousal disorders and many other clinical situations. Tricyclics such as desipramine and amitriptyline have been used in this age group, but not as widely as imipramine (Table 2).

Tricyclic antidepressants may have several different mechanisms of action in the CNS and elsewhere that result in their effectiveness in these several different conditions. In general, the tricyclics prevent reuptake of catecholamines or indoleamines at the receptor level in the CNS, and have both adrenergic and anticholinergic activity in the CNS and PNS. Enuretic and hyperactive children tend to respond to imipramine within days of beginning drug therapy, whereas school refusers and depressed children tend to require several weeks to respond.

Studies seem to indicate that imipramine's effectiveness in enuresis is not related to its anticholinergic properties nor to its effects on sleep architecture but perhaps through some direct effects on bladder muscles (20).

The mechanism of action in school refusers has not been clearly elucidated at this time. In one placebo-controlled study (21), 35 school-age children who had failed to return to school through behavioral means returned with imipramine treatment on the average of 159 mg/day. This study has not been replicated, however.

Table 2A. Antidepressants for Use in Children Over 12 Years of Age

Generic Name (Trade Name)	Indications	Dosage Range (mg)	Common Side Effects	
			Short-Term	Long-Term
Imipramine (Tofranil)[a]	Enuresis;	25–125 (imipramine)	Autonomic Nervous System: dry mouth, orthostatic hypotension, urinary retention, blurring vision CNS: seizures, precipitate mania/psychosis Cardiovascular: alterations in conduction, pulse, blood pressure; prolonged PR, QRS; arrhythmias	Same as short-term
	hyperactivity/attention deficit disorder;	25–200 (imipramine)		
	Depression	100–300 (imipramine)		
	Separation anxiety (school refusal)	100–200 (imipramine)		

Others
Amitriptyline (Elavil)
Desipramine (Norpramin)
Nortriptyline (Aventyl)
Doxepin (Sinequan)
Maprotiline (Ludiomil)
Amoxapine (Asendin)[c]
Trazodone (Desyrel)[b]

---

[a]FDA approved for advertising for use in children over 6 years old for enuresis, over 12 years old for depression.
[b]FDA approved for advertising for use in children over 18 years old.
[c]FDA approved for advertising for use in children over 16 years old.

Table 2B. Recommended Antidepressant Treatment

Suggested Treatment Regimen for Enuresis
- Start with 0.5 mg/kg of imipramine for 2–3 nights
- Increase by 25 or 0.5 mg/kg every 2–3 nights until therapeutic response
- Daily maintenance dose range: 0.5–2.5 mg/kg

Suggested Treatment Regimen for Hyperactivity and Attention Deficit Disorder
- Start with 0.5 mg/kg imipramine
- Increase by 25 or 0.5 mg/kg every 5–7 days until therapeutic response or side effects
- Daily maintenance dose range: 0.5–3.0 mg/kg

Suggested Treatment Regimen for Childhood Depression
- Start with 0.5 mg/kg imipramine for 2–3 days
- Increase by 0.5 mg/kg every 3–4 days
- Daily maintenance dose range: 3–5 mg/kg

There has been increasing interest in recent years in childhood depression and evidence has accumulated that adolescents and even prepubertal children can meet adult research criteria or *DSM-III* criteria for major depression.

Studies have shown (22) that some of these children are responsive to tricyclic antidepressant treatment in fairly high dose ranges, 3 to 5 mg/kg.

Newer antidepressants such as trazodone and maprotiline have had some informal use in this country, but no controlled studies in this age group have been performed to date.

Experience in this country with monoamine oxidase (MAO) inhibitors in this age group is extremely limited, particularly in the prepubertal child. Due to their potential for toxicity, these are difficult to prescribe for most youngsters. Some adolescents with atypical depressive features or phobias may be candidates.

Side effects of tricyclic antidepressants are primarily anticholinergic, cardiovascular, and CNS. Lowering of seizure threshold is of significant concern. Cardiovascular effects include increased pulse, blood pressure, PR interval, and arrhythmias. Serial EKG monitoring should take place above 3.5 mg/kg/day.

Anxiolytics and Sedative–Hypnotics

Despite widespread use in pediatric practice, anxiolytics and sedative–hypnotics have not been well studied in this population. Due to their safety and nonspecificity of action, these medications have been used for a number of childhood and adolescent conditions such as night terrors, insomnia, anxiety, and hyperactivity.

There are two major classes of medication in this category that are useful in a number of clinical situations: 1) antihistamines such as diphenhydramine and hydroxyzine and 2) benzodiazepines such as diazepam and chlordiazepoxide (Table 3). Experience with other sedative–hypnotics such as barbiturates and propanediols for anxiolysis is limited in this age group.

The mechanism of action of the antihistamines is thought

Table 3A. Anxiolytics and Sedative-Hypnotics for Use in Children Over 6 Years of Age

Generic Name (Trade Name)	Indications	Dosage Range (mg)	Common Side Effects Short-Term	Common Side Effects Long-Term
Antihistamines				
Diphenhydramine (Benadryl)[a]	Bedtime sedation	25–500	Oversedation, hypersensitivity; skin rash, dryness of mucous membranes	
Hydroxyzine (Vistaril or Atarax)[a]	Anxiety states, agitation, bedtime sedation	25–500		
Benzodiazepines				
Diazepam (Valium)[a]	Night terrors; exogenous anxiety	1–20 2–10	Drowsiness Paradoxical agitation or excitement	
Chlordiazepoxide (Librium)		10–100		Withdrawal reactions
Alprazolam (Xanax)[b]	Separation anxiety	0.25–5		
Flurazepam (Dalmane)[c]	Bedtime sedation	15–30	Daytime sedation	
Other				
Chloral Hydrate (Noctec)[a]	Bedtime sedation	500–1000		

[a]FDA approved for advertising for use in children under 6 years old.
[b]FDA approved for advertising for use in children over 18 years old.
[c]FDA approved for advertising for use in children over 15 years old.

Table 3B. Recommended Anxiolytic and Sedative-Hypnotic Treatment

Suggested Treatment Regimens for Sleep Induction (children over 6 years old)
Diphenhydramine or Hydroxyzine
- Start with 25–50 mg at bedtime, increase every 2 days by 25 mg until therapeutic effect
- Daily maintenance range 25–500 mg at bedtime or 2.0 to 5.0 mg/kg

Chloral Hydrate
- 500 to 1000 mg at bedtime

Suggested Treatment Regimen for Pavor Nocturnus (Night Terrors)
Diazepam
- Start at 1 mg at bedtime, then increase by 0.5 mg every 2–4 days until therapeutic response
- Daily maintenance dose range 1–20 mg at bedtime

Suggested Treatment Regimens for Anxiety/Agitation:
Diphenhydramine or Hydroxyzine
- Acute: Start with 25–50 mg, then repeat dose every 2–4 hours until therapeutic effect
- Nonacute: Start with 25–50 mg, then increase by 25 mg every 2–3 days
- Daily maintenance dose range: 75–500 mg or up to 5 mg/kg/day

Chlordiazepoxide
- Start with 5–10 mg, then increase by 5–10 mg every 3–4 days until response
- Daily maintenance dose range: 45–90 mg

to be blockade of the central muscarinic action of acetylcholine, and blockade of H1 histamine receptors.

The antihistamines are useful for anxiolysis in the nonpsychotic, mild to moderately disturbed population of children and for sedation/hypnotic effects in the preschool through adolescent age groups. Sleep disturbances such as inability to fall asleep due to restlessness, fearfulness, or hyperactivity in the young child are likely to respond to an antihistamine.

Night terrors (pavor nocturnus) is a particular form of sleep disturbance seen in young children during N-REM sleep, frequently on arousal from Stage 3 or 4 to lighter sleep stages. Characteristically, the child awakens in a terror, screaming, with signs of physiological arousal, and is unconsolable during the episode for which the child is amnestic. Diazepam in small doses administered at bedtime for several weeks can be useful for this particular problem.

Benzodiazepines have been found to be generally safe and effective anxiolytics for adult patients. There are few studies of such use in the pediatric population in this country. They seem to function as "selective depressants" possibly acting on subcortical structures or specific receptors. There have been some reports of paradoxical reactions or disinhibition to these drugs in young patients, such as pathological aggression or excitement; perhaps this has limited their practical use and investigation. Another dilemma for the pediatric practitioner has been the confusion and lack of validated criteria for defining "anxiety" and its manifestations in this age group.

In the nonpsychotic, nonsubstance-using adolescent population, benzodiazepines can be useful in limited quantities for anxiety that threatens to interfere with daily functioning. Chlordiazepoxide and diazepam have found some usefulness in this situation. In some adolescents with early and middle insomnia, flurazepam can be used for limited periods of time.

Chloral hydrate is also a safe and effective nighttime sedative for this population. Interest has increased recently in the use of a newer anxiolytic, alprazolam, in the child and adolescent with separation anxiety–panic disorder symptomatology, paralleling its uses in adults with endogenous anxiety.

Side effects with both of these classes of medication are relatively infrequent, particularly with the antihistamines.

Lithium

Interest in and experience with lithium in the child and adolescent population has increased significantly in the past several years.

While lithium has been clearly found to be effective for treatment of acute mania and prophylaxis for bipolar disorders in the adult population, these disorders are infrequently found in the pediatric population in the adult form. Nevertheless, studies suggest that some adolescents and children with certain kinds of behavior disorders can be treated effectively with lithium despite lack of formal indications for use in this age group (Table 4).

It appears that children with periodic or cyclic disturbances of behavior and mood, children with such disturbances who have relatives who have been lithium responsive, and children with severely aggressive behavior disorders are potentially lithium responsive (23–25). Studies are ongoing in this area at the present time, and promise a potentially exciting and useful approach to some of the most difficult patients in the child psychiatric population.

The mechanism of action of lithium is not completely clear. Some theories have proposed effects on neurotransmitters, cyclic adenosine monophosphate, or membrane stabilization.

Because children and adolescents run the same risks for side effects and toxicities as do their adult counterparts, they must be carefully worked up and monitored. Children and adolescents frequently need higher doses of lithium than adults, relative to body weight.

Plasma levels should be obtained in order to monitor clinical effects on a regular basis. During initiation of treatment, twice weekly levels are called for, which can be followed by weekly and then approximately monthly levels once equilibrium and steady state has been reached. Levels of 0.6 to 1.6 mEq/L are in therapeutic range, but some patients may require up to 1.8–2.0 mEq/L to attain therapeutic efficacy. Kidney, en-

Table 4A. Lithium for Use in Children Over 12 Years of Age

Generic Name (Trade Name)	Indications	Dosage Range (mg)	Common Side Effects Short-Term	Common Side Effects Long-Term
Lithium carbonate (Eskalith or Lithobid)[a]	Bipolar and some recurrent unipolar affective disorders; some behavior disorders	150+	Gastrointestinal: nausea, vomiting, diarrhea, abominal distress	
			CNS: tremor, memory lapses, fatigue	
			Renal: polyurea, polydipsia, tubular changes	Same
			Hematologic: leukocytosis	
			Endocrine: goiter	Same

[a] FDA approved for advertising for use in children over 12 years old.

Table 4B. Recommended Lithium Treatment

Suggested Treatment Regimen for Childhood and Adolescent Bipolar/Periodic Disorders and Aggressive Behavior (Children Over 6 Years of Age)

- Start with 150 mg in the a.m., then increase by 150 mg q 3–4 days until blood level in 0.8–1.5 mEq/L range (some adolescents may require higher doses approaching 2.0 mEq/L)
- Daily maintenance dose range: 300–2400 mg daily

Table 5. Anticonvulsant Medications for Use in Children

Generic Name (Trade Name)	Dosage (mg/kg/day)	Therapeutic Serum Concentration (µg/ml)	Type of Seizures	Common Side Effects
Carbamazepine (Tegretol)	10–30	4–12	All except petit mal and infantile spasms, especially valuable in complex partial seizures	Dose-Related: drowsiness, ataxia, dysarthria Other: gastrointestinal upset, leukopenia, thrombocytopenia, elevation of liver enzymes
Clonazepam (Clonopin)	0.01–0.15	0.015–0.06	Petit mal, minor motor; adjunctive therapy in major motor	Dose-related: sedation, dizziness Other: behavioral effects including impulsivity, irritability, sleep disturbance, inattentiveness
Chlorazepate (Tranxene)	0.3–1.0	0.05–0.075	Adjunctive therapy for generalized & partial seizures, especially complex partial	Dose-related: sedation, dizziness Other: elevation of liver enzymes, gastrointestinal distress
Ethosuccimide (Zarontin)	20–40	40–120	Petit mal; adjunctive for refractory seizures	Dose-related: sedation Other: nausea, vomiting, irritability, sleep disturbance, leukopenia, pancytopenia
Phenobarbital	2–6	20–40	All except petit mal and infantile spasms	Dose-related: sedation, ataxia, irritability Other: hyperactivity, irritability, depressed affect, attention deficit disorder, hypocalcemia
Phenytoin (Dilantin)	5–10	10–20	All except petit mal and infantile spasms	Dose-related: nystagmus, ataxia, irritability Other: irritability, depressed affect, gum hypertrophy, hirsuitism, tremor, fever, lymphadenopathy, choreoathetosis, thickened facial features
Primidone (Mysoline)	10–20	5–15[a]	All except petit mal and infantile spasms; especially valuable for complex partial and myocloric	Dose-related: sedation, ataxia, irritability Other: hyperactivity, irritability, depressed affect, attention deficit disorder, hypocalcemia

Table 5. (Continued)

Generic Name (Trade Name)	Dosage (mg/kg/day)	Therapeutic Serum Concentration (µg/ml)	Type of Seizures	Common Side Effects
Mephobarbital (meberal)	6–12	20–40[b] (measured as phenobarbital)	All except petit mal and infantile spasms	See phenobarbital
Valproic acid (Depakene)	30–60	50–150	Petit mal and refractory major and minor motor	Dose-related: sedation, elevation of liver enzymes Other: nausea, vomiting, tremor, transient hair loss, leukopenia, thrombocytopenia, pancreatitis, hepatotoxicity[c]
Progabide	20–30	0.050–0.075	Refractory generalized and partial complex	Dose-related: sedation Other: leukopenia, elevated liver enzymes, gastrointestinal irritation
Phenacemide (Phenurone)	25–40	Not usually measured	All refractory seizures except petit mal and infantile spasms	Dose-related: sedation Other: personality disorders including suicide attempt, psychosis, depression, and aggression; hepatitis, leukopenia, aplastic anemia
Acetazolamide (Diamox)	10–20	Not usually measured	Adjunct in petit mal and major motor	Dose-related: sedation, gastric distress Other: crystaluria, renal calculus, bone marrow depression, hemolytic anemia, thrombocytopenia purpura, drowsiness, confusion

[a]Primidone is metabolized in part to phenobarbital and phenylethylmalonamide; only primidone and phenobarbital are usually measured.
[b]Measured as phenobarbital.
[c]Hypersensitivity and drug allergy may occur with any anticonvulsant.

docrine, and cardiac function must be monitored on a regular basis.

Anticonvulsants

Knowledge of and familiarity with anticonvulsant medication is a necessity for the practicing child psychiatrist. Psychiatric symptoms and psychopathology appear to be overrepresented in epileptic patients; seizures themselves are often accompanied by changes in mood or behavior. Patients with temporal lobe epilepsy are frequently complicated, requiring the skills of a psychiatrist and neurologist working together.

Seizures can be roughly divided into the following types:

Partial
1. with simple focal symptoms: motor or sensory (no clouding of consciousness)
2. with complex symptoms: temporal lobe, psychomotor seizures (clouding of consciousness)

Generalized (clouding of consciousness)
1. tonic-clonic seizures
2. myoclonic, atonic, or akinetic seizures
3. absence or petit mal

Anticonvulsants can be roughly divided into the following groups: hydantoins, barbiturates, carbamazepine, succinimides, benzodiazepines, sodium valproate, and others.

Table 5 outlines anticonvulsants commonly used for different types of seizures, their dosage ranges, and common side effects.

The Use of Antiparkinsonian Agents

The psychopharmacologic treatment of extrapyramidal symptoms as side effects of neuroleptic therapy in childhood follows guidelines used for adults.

In general, except for the acute dystonic reactions, it is best to try to decrease neuroleptic dosage before adding an antiparkinsonian agent. If decreasing neuroleptic dosage is not possible, then antiparkinsonian treatment is indicated.

In general, our practice is to avoid prophylactic antiparkinsonian medication despite the controversy in the literature. In our experience, choosing a neuroleptic less likely to cause EPS and using lowest possible maintenance dosages lessens the possibility of EPS development. Should the symptoms develop, however, an antiparkinsonian agent can be readily added.

In the case of acute dystonic reaction, treatment with intramuscular diphenhydramine or benztropine mesylate is indicated. The child can then be maintained on p.o. forms for 2 to 4 weeks and then have it discontinued. Any recurrence of EPS symptomatology is indication for further treatment.

For dosages, see Table 6.

Other Drugs

In recent years, other drugs available to the adult practitioner have gained informal or experimental usage in the pediatric and adolescent population. The β-adrenergic blocker propranolol has found use in some young patients with uncontrollable aggressive behavior (26), those with lithium-induced tremors, and those with certain anxiety states manifest by physiological symptomatology. They are contraindicated in diabetics, asthmatics, and patients with cardiac disease.

Table 6. Antiparkinsonian Medications for Use in Children Over 3 Years of Age

Generic Name	(Trade Name)	Indications	Dosage Range (mg)
Diphenhydramine[a]	(Benadryl)	Acute dystonic reactions	25–50 i.m.
Benztropine Mesylate	(Cogentin)	EPS: parkinsonism akathisia	1–2 i.m. 1–6 p.o. daily
Trihexyphenidyl	(Artane)		2–6 p.o. daily

[a]FDA approved for advertising for use in children over 3 years old.

Table 7. Side Effects and Their Management in Children and Adolescents

Drug Category	Common Adverse Effects	Clinical Management
Neuroleptics (Antipsychotics)	**Short-Term** Autonomic Nervous System • Dry mouth	In general, lower dosage if possible or switch drug if persistent; child may "equilibrate" after several weeks Bethanecol only if severe and persistent
	• Urinary retention • Constipation	Dioctyl sodium sulfosuccinate (Colace) tablets or bisacodyl USP (Dulcolax) suppositories
	• Orthostatic hypotension Extrapyramidal • Acute dystonic reaction	Avoid sudden postural changes; dosage reduction if severe Diphenhydramine or benzotropine (i.m.), then switch to oral form
	• Parkinsonism	Anticholinergic/antiparkinsonian medication on an as needed basis
	Other • Akathisia • Hypersensitivity/rash • Drowsiness	Lower dosage; sometimes anticholinergic can help Discontinue drug Child usually becomes tolerant; if persistent switch to less sedating class
	• Photosensitivity • LFTs	Avoid sun exposure May not have clinical significance
	Long-Term • Weight gain • Dyskinesias (tardive and withdrawal)	Lower dosage; consider switch to another class Prevention is best; use lowest possible dose for maintenance
Psychostimulants	**Short-Term** • Anorexia, nausea, abdominal pain	Reduce dose; give most of dosage in the a.m.; consider switch

Table 7. (Continued)

Drug Category	Common Adverse Effects	Clinical Management
	• Insomnia	Move p.m. dose to earlier in the day; reduce dosage; then reintroduce
	• Dysphoria	Consider another stimulant if persistent or imipramine
	Long-Term	
	• Weight loss	Institute drug holidays or change drug
	• Tics/Tourette's	Discontinue immediately and avoid rechallenge
Tricyclic Antidepressants	Autonomic Nervous System	See neuroleptics
	Cardiovascular (blood pressure, pulse, PR, T-wave changes, and arrhythmias)	Monitor EKGs serially with dosages 3.5 mg/kg; most changes have little clinical significance in healthy child
	CNS (seizures)	Discontinue medication gradually; EEG; may need anticonvulsant
Anxiolytics-Sedative Hypnotics		
Antihistamines	Oversedation	Decrease total dosage, administer most at bedtime
	Rash	Discontinue medication
Benzodiazepines	Disinhibition	Discontinue medication
	Gastrointestinal: nausea, vomiting, abdominal pain, diarrhea, metallic taste	Consider dose reduction if persistent
	CNS: tremor, memory lapses, fatigue	Consider dose reduction if persistent
Lithium	Endocrine: goiter	Discontinue medication and follow with lab studies
	Renal: polyuria/polydipsia	Monitor BUN, creatinine, electrolytes, and urinalysis on a regular basis (q 2–3 months)
	Hematologic: leukocytosis	Monitor; may not be of clinical significance

Their use is still experimental in this age group at this time.

The α-agonist clonidine has enjoyed increasing clinical use and has been found in some studies to be a useful adjunct to treatment of Tourette's syndrome. It can be used in combination with haloperidol in low doses or as a primary drug therapy. Some evidence indicates that it has been useful for the motor and verbal tics that characterize the disorder, as well as useful in modifying the behavioral concomitants that often accompany the tics such as attentional problems, hyperactivity, and lability of mood (27).

Blood pressure and pulse must be closely monitored during treatment.

Management of Side Effects and Toxic Effects

Despite their drug handling efficiency, children and adolescents are no less at risk for the development of adverse effects of these agents (Table 7). This has both physiologic and practical significance: The clinician must be acquainted with the side effect profiles of the drug(s) being prescribed and must know how to manage adverse effects should they arise. In addition, children and adolescents are particularly prone to sensitivities about their bodies and how they work, and often get quite frightened or suspicious if a sudden change or dysfunction occurs in the context of drug therapy. Such feelings can interfere with compliance.

In general, the best therapy for adverse effects is preventive. The following are *guidelines* to avoid possible adverse effects:

- Use the lowest possible maintenance doses in the therapeutic range once it has been established.
- Try to avoid prescribing more than one drug at a time in a given child. For example, it is best to try lowering the dosage of a neuroleptic slightly for parkinsonism or akathisia if at all possible, rather than adding an antiparkinsonian agent.

- In most cases, drugs should be tapered gradually to discontinue them, both for physiologic and psychologic purposes. This provides more opportunity for the reestablishment of equilibrium.
- Avoid giving an agent to a child who has demonstrated previous sensitivity to it such as tics with stimulants or dyskinesias with phenothiazines.

COMMON DRUG INTERACTIONS IN CHILDREN AND ADOLESCENTS

Drug interaction occurs when one agent alters the therapeutic or adverse effects of another agent. Interactions can occur at any phase in a drug treatment plan. Common points of interaction include:

- Alterations in *absorption*, such as in the gastrointestinal tract;
- Alterations in *distribution*, such as competition for binding sites
- Alterations in *metabolism*, such as effects on liver enzyme functions
- Alterations in *excretion*
- Alterations in *receptor site* function (2)

Children and adolescents are no less prone to drug interaction effects than are adults. The best rule of thumb is to try to avoid interactive effects by avoiding polypharmacy where at all possible. However, if at times it becomes necessary to prescribe two or more agents simultaneously, the clinician should be alert to possible interactions.

A few of the more common drug interactions to occur in childhood are listed in Table 8.

Table 8. Common Drug Interactions in Children and Adolescents

	Neuroleptics	Stimulants	Antidepressants	Sedative/Hypnotics/Anxiolytics	Lithium
Neuroleptics	—	See under neuroleptics	See under neuroleptics; can raise TCA blood levels	See under neuroleptics	Neuroleptics can suppress nausea 2° to lithium toxicity
Stimulants	Thioridazine raises MPH effects in hyperactives	—	See under stimulants	See under stimulants	—
Antidepressants	TCAs potentiate anticholinergic effects; both lower seizure threshold	MPH raises effects of TCAs and raises blood levels; MAOI and stimulants to be avoided	TCA-MAOI combination problematic	Potentiate anticholinergic effects of MAOI	—
Sedative/Hypnotics/Anxiolytics	Neuroleptics potentiate CNS depressants	Stimulants may oppose hypnotic effects	—	—	—
Lithium	Some reports of neuroleptic-haloperidol neurotoxicity	—	—	—	—

Table 8. (Continued)

	Neuroleptics	Stimulants	Antidepressants	Sedative/Hypnotics/Anxiolytics	Lithium
Others: Anticonvulsants	Can raise sedation but not anticonvulsant effect	—	Barbiturates lower TCA blood levels	—	—
Anticoagulants	Phenothiazine lowers effect	MPH potentiates effect of ethyl bis-coumacetate	—	Chloral hydrate lowers effects of coumarin preparations	—
Antiinflamatory Agents	—	MPH inhibits action of phenylbutazone	—	—	—
Vasopressors	Neuroleptics block effect of Epinephrine and lower blood pressure	—	—	—	—
Antihelminitics	Piperazine and phenothiazines cause seizures	—	—	—	—
Diuretics	Can lower blood pressure	—	—	—	Lowers lithium clearance and raises lithium toxicity

TCA = tricyclic antidepressants. MAOI = monoamine oxidase inhibitor.

REFERENCES

1. American Psychiatric Association: Diagnostic and Statistical Manual of Mental Disorders, Third Edition. Washington, DC, American Psychiatric Association, 1980

2. Briant RH: An introduction to clinical pharmacology, in Pediatric Psychopharmacology: The Use of Behavior Modifying Drugs in Childhood. Edited by Werry J. New York, Brunner/Mazel, 1978, pp 3–28

3. Rapaport J, Mikkelson E: Antidepressants, in Pediatric Psychopharmacology: The Use of Behavior Modifying Drugs in Childhood. Edited by Werry J. New York, Brunner/Mazel, 1978, pp 208–233

4. Popper C, Famularo R: Child and adolescent psychopharmacology, in Developmental-Behavioral Pediatrics. Edited by Levine MD, Carey WB. Philadelphia, W. B. Saunders, 1983, pp 1138–1159

5. Klein D, Gittelman R, Quitkin F, et al: Diagnosis and Drug Treatment of Psychiatric Disorders: Adults and Children, 2nd ed. Baltimore, Williams & Wilkins, 1980

6. Gualtieri T, et al: Tardive dyskinesia and other movement disorders in children treated with psychotropic drugs. J Am Acad Child Psychiatry 19:491–510, 1980

7. Campbell M, Gregs D, et al: Neuroleptic-induced dyskinesias in children. Clin Neuropharmacol 6:207–222, 1983

8. U.S. Department of Human Services, Alcohol and Drug Abuse and Mental Health Administration: Abnormal Involuntary Movement Screen. Rockville, Md, National Institute of Mental Health, 1974

9. Conners CK: Rating scales for use in drug studies with children, in Assessment Manual (Early Clinical Drug Evaluation Unit). Rockville, Md, National Institute of Mental Health, 1976

10. Growth Chart. Washington, DC, U.S. Department of Human Services, Health Resources Administration, National Center for Health Statistics, Centers for Disease Control, 1978

11. Campbell M, Shapiro T: Therapy of psychiatric disorders of childhood, in Manual of Psychiatric Therapeutics. Edited by Shader RI. Boston, Little, Brown, 1975, pp 137–162

12. Polizos P, Englehardt P, Hoffman SP: Neurological consequences of psychotropic drug withdrawal in schizophrenic children. J Autism Child Schiz 3:247–253, 1973

13. Gualtieri CT, Quade D, Hicks R, et al: Tardive dyskinesia and other clinical consequences of neuroleptic treatment in children and adolescents. Am J Psychiatry 141:20–23, 1984

14. Cantwell D, Carlson G: Stimulants, in Pediatric Psychopharmacology: The Use of Behavior Modifying Drugs in Childhood. Edited by Werry J. New York, Brunner/Mazel, 1978, pp 171–207

15. Rapaport J, Buschbaum M, et al: Dextroamphetamine: its cognitive and behavioral effects in normal and hyperactive boys and normal men. Arch Gen Psychiatry 37:933–943, 1980

16. Cohen D, Shaywitz B, Shaywitz S, et al: Pharmacotherapy of attention deficit disorders, in Pediatric Update, Vol. 5. Edited by Moss AJ. New York, Elsevier-North Holland, 1983, pp 43–61

17. Sprague R, Sleator E: Methylphenidate in hyperkinetic children: differences in dose effects in learning and social behavior. Science 198:1274–1276, 1977

18. Safer D, Allen R, et al: Depression of growth in hyperactive children on stimulant drugs. N Engl J Med 287:217–220, 1972

19. Mattes J, Gittelman R: Growth of hyperactive children on maintenance regimen of methylphenidate. Arch Gen Psychiatry 40:317–321, 1983

20. Rapaport J, Mikkelsen E, et al: Childhood enuresis I and II. Arch Gen Psychiatry 37:1139–1152, 1980

21. Gittleman-Klein R: Pharmacotherapy and management of pathological separation anxiety. International Journal of Mental Health 4:255–271, 1975

22. Puig-Antich J: Affective disorders in childhood: a review and perspective. Psychiatr Clin North Am 3:403–424, 1980
23. DeLong R: Lithium carbonate treatment of select behavior disorders in children suggesting manic-depressive illness. J Pediatr 93:689–699, 1977
24. Youngerman J, Cannino I: Lithium carbonate use in children and adolescents. Arch Gen Psychiatry 35:216–224, 1978
25. Campbell M, Cohen I, Small A: Drugs in aggressive behavior. J Am Acad Child Psychiatry 21:107–117, 1982
26. Williams D, Meyl R, Yudofsky S, et al: The effects of propranolol on uncontrolled rage outbursts in children and adolescents with organic brain dysfunction. J Am Acad Child Psychiatry 21:129–135, 1982
27. Cohen D, Detlor J, et al: Clonidine ameliorates Gilles de la Tourette syndrome. Arch Gen Psychiatry 37:1350–1357, 1980

Chapter 10

Emergencies I

Judith Robinson, M.D.

When a child is brought to the emergency room for psychiatric consultation, the child's *physical safety* represents the first priority of the consulting psychiatrist. It is the psychiatrist's responsibility to assess the nature of the presenting problem rapidly and to determine what *immediate course of action* needs to be taken. The psychiatrist must decide if the child:

- needs medical intervention by the pediatrician on call,
- requires constant observation for suicidal precautions,
- is at risk for running away from the emergency room, or
- is at risk of being taken prematurely from the emergency room by a caretaker.

Only when the child's physical safety has been assured can a systematic evaluation process begin.

A *thorough psychiatric examination* is essential for the successful management of psychiatric emergencies. Such data provide the child psychiatrist with the information necessary to make a working formulation, an accurate diagnosis, and an appropriate treatment plan. In the emergency room, as in the clinic, a complete evaluation includes the following:

- Presenting problem
- Present illness and precipitating stress
- Family history and composition (with special attention to present stresses and the ability of the family to cope with the child now)
- Developmental history (as relevant)
- Medical history (as relevant)
- Detailed interview with the child and family, including mental status examination.

The physical examination should be part of every evaluation, particularly if the child presents with suspected or confirmed physical or sexual abuse, alcohol or drug abuse or overdose, abrupt change in behavior, or suicidal attempts.

Additional information may need to be gathered from sources other than the child or the parents. Such sources often include the child's therapist, social service worker, or pediatrician. Ready access in the emergency room to frequently used telephone numbers facilitates the evaluation.

In evaluating psychiatric emergencies in childhood, an assessment must also be made of the child's parent or caretaker. This is important because psychiatric illness in childhood reflects the interplay between the child's psychopathology and that of the caretaker. In cases of sexual or physical abuse, in particular, the psychopathology may reside more with the caretaker than with the child.

SUICIDE

Suicidal ideation and behavior are among the most frequent psychiatric emergencies in childhood and adolescence.

Although successfully completed suicide is virtually nonexistent in children under 5 and rare in children 6 to 12, the suicide rate in adolescence is significant and is rapidly increasing. In the 15- to 24-year-old age group, suicide is the third leading cause of death. Girls attempt suicide three times as frequently as boys; however, boys complete suicide two to three times as frequently as girls (1, 2).

Any child who attempts suicide usually does so as a last resort. Even if the suicidal behavior is seen as a gesture and not as a genuine effort to end life, it must *always* be seen as a desperate attempt on the part of the child and must *always* be taken seriously. It is important to remember that a proportion of children who attempt suicide later go on to complete suicide. A suicidal gesture is a psychiatric emergency.

Suicidal ideation and behavior in childhood usually reflect serious and chronic problems within the family. Children who contemplate suicide have frequently had early separation from their parents or inadequate mothering, sometimes including physical and emotional abuse. Often these children present as depressed, empty, and lonely, with an accompanying sense of themselves as expendable.

Often the child of latency age or younger may threaten or attempt suicide without understanding the nature of death, its permanence, and its irreversibility. For children of this age death may mean removal from an unpleasant situation to a happier one; it may also be an attempt to gain love from unresponsive parents or to join a parent or loved one who has died.

In a recent study of suicidal behavior in children ages 6 to 12, Pfeffer et al. (3) found that a child's suicidal potential correlated significantly with a sense of depression, hopelessness, and worthlessness; with parents' depression and suicidal behavior; and with a belief that death is temporary and pleasant.

Suicidal adolescents understand the meaning of death. Usually these youngsters are seriously troubled. They frequently present with depression or with antisocial behavior (turning their aggression outward as a defense against their depression). Most have very low self-esteem. Prior to their suicide attempts there may be difficulties in other areas of life (such as failure in school, trouble with the law, or the end of a romantic relationship) that further lower self-esteem. The adolescent may feel overwhelmed and desperate. Most suicide attempts represent the child's or adolescent's effort at extrication from an impossible situation resulting either from internal or external stress.

Evaluation

The immediate treatment of a suicide attempt is to provide medical lifesaving measures. Only when the patient is out of danger can the formal evaluative process begin.

The suicidal patient should be evaluated in a safe environment and should be seen in a room with no sharp objects and no open windows. At no time should the patient be left alone.

The child psychiatric consultant must establish a working alliance with the child or adolescent. In a nonjudgmental and nonpunitive manner, the consultant must stress the seriousness of the situation and convey genuine concern and desire to help. Ideally the child and family should be interviewed separately and the child should be helped to understand clearly that his or her feelings are important and will be listened to.

The evaluation should follow the format outlined earlier in this chapter, with special attention to the following:

Presenting Problem. It is important to assess

- *The lethality* of the suicidal attempt or action. What did the patient do to try to commit suicide, what was the likelihood of success, was the action planned or impulsive, was the rescue imminent, was a note left?
- *The motivation.* Why does the patient want to commit suicide, is the patient angry with someone, does the patient want to gain the love of someone or to join a dead relative, is the suicidal action in response to any hallucination, what does it mean to the patient to be dead, what does the patient think that it will mean to important others for him or her to be dead?
- *Current attitude.* What does it mean to the patient *not* to have died, is the patient sad or glad, are there plans to try again? These data are particularly good indicators of the acute risk of further suicidal behavior (4).

The Precipitating Stress. It is important to ask specifically about

- The child's relationship with parents or caretakers, emphasizing any recent arguments or problems.
- Any changes within the family, any illnesses, any losses (or anniversaries of losses).
- Any break-up in a romantic relationship or an important friendship.
- Any difficulties in school, any problem with the authorities, any situation in which the parents may soon learn something very negative about the child.
- Any change that may have altered the patient's view of life or of self-worth.
- Participation in incest or sexual abuse.

Interview with the Family. An essential element of the psychiatric evaluation is the interview with the parents or caretakers. A suicide attempt on the part of the child is a *family* problem, and most suicidal children have a history of long-standing family problems. It is important to assess the family's conscious and unconscious attitude toward the patient and toward the patient's suicide attempt.

Continued suicide risk is associated with

- A negative attitude or lack of concern toward the patient.
- A minimization of the seriousness and an attempt to see it only as attention-getting behavior.
- The family's stability and their desire and ability to cope with the child and provide a safe, supportive environment.
- The incidence in the family of suicide attempts, and serious depression, because suicidal attempts in children correspond significantly with parental suicidal ideation (3).

Mental Status Exam. It is critical to assess the patient's reality testing, judgment, impulse control, mood, and affect. It is essential to determine if the patient's suicidal ideation is based on a psychiatric disorder such as psychosis (are voices telling the patient to commit suicide), affective illness, or intoxication with alcohol or drugs.

After the child and family have been interviewed and pertinent historical information has been gathered, a psychodynamic formulation must be made. This formulation should help to clarify what forces have combined to place this particular child in jeopardy and make his or her life not worth living, and what changes are necessary to shift the equilibrium. The child psychiatrist must determine whether these changes are possible given information on the child and the child's family and situation.

Assessment. Final assessment of the suicidal child should take into account that certain children are statistically at high risk for self-destructive behavior. These include children

- with chronic family problems
- living outside of a natural family
- with poor relationships and few supports
- with poor school performance
- with family history of suicide attempts
- whose parents do not like them or whose parents see them as expendable
- with a concomitant psychiatric diagnosis or a history of drug or alcohol abuse
- who understand the meaning of death and who have a true wish to die
- whose attempt was very lethal
- who make poor relationships with the evaluator
- who have made a previous suicide attempt
- who are depressed and hopeless

Disposition of a Suicidal Child or Adolescent

The primary goal of the child psychiatric consultant is to keep the child safe from harm. The question that inevitably arises in the emergency room is whether the child is safe to go home or whether hospitalization is needed. The decision depends on a variety of factors:

- The child's *immediate potential* for continued self-destructive behavior.
- *Concurrent psychopathology* of the child. If the child is psychotic, hypomanic, severely depressed, or intoxicated with drugs or alcohol, the child must be held in the protective environment of the hospital.
- The assessment of the child's *intrapsychic needs*, based on the psychodynamic formulation and the likelihood that these needs can be adequately met. If they cannot be met, in short order, the child must be held in the protective environment.
- The *family's unambivalent desire* for the *child* to *live*, their understanding of the suicidal behavior as an individual as well as a family problem, their ability to mobilize around the child and to assume appropriate parental response for the child. Since most suicidal children have chronic and complicated family problems, parents may not be able to make immediate changes that are necessary and the child may need psychiatric hospitalization as the initial treatment (5).
- *Practical limitations* of the family's ability to provide supervised support and keep the patient safe from harm.

If there is any doubt as to whether or not the patient should be sent home from the emergency room, the child should be hospitalized. Within the hospital, protection from physical harm continues to be the primary concern. The suicidal child should be placed in a safe room without sharp objects or access to windows through which the child could exit. Around-the-clock sitters who can observe and protect the child or other suicidal precautions will be required, depending on the setting's structure. For the severely agitated or psychotic child, chemical or physical restraints may be necessary.

In the event that the child is sent home, a follow-up appointment should be made for the next day, and a phone number should be given to the family member for emergency contact.

AGGRESSION

Many children are brought to the emergency room with the presenting problem of aggressive behavior. In most situations of this kind, by the time the psychiatrist sees the patient, the presenting behavior has subsided and evaluation is based largely on historical information.

Extreme aggressive behavior in preschool children (who are medically and neurologically intact) is usually reflective of child–parent problems. This is especially true when the parents report the aggressive behavior as directed primarily toward them. Often these are children with whom the parents have an ambivalent attachment; such children are frequently raised with little limit-setting, at times by a parent who is masochistic. Many of these children may act out their parent's unconscious hostility. In other instances, the child may come from a family where aggression and physical acting out is the norm. In this case the child's aggressive behavior may reflect both the heightening of aggressive drives and an identification with an aggressive parent.

Aggression seen in older children usually reflects unhappiness and insecurity. Aggressive behavior frequently is seen in response to frustation related particularly to problems with alcohol, peers, or family members who are seen as uncaring.

In the adolescent, aggressive behavior usually follows a build-up of tension. Often a struggle over control precipitates an episode of rage. Threats may be made, doors may be slammed, chairs may be thrown, but usually no one is hurt, and by the time the adolescent is seen the anger has dissipated.

In most instances, the consultant's task is crisis intervention. After evaluating the situation, listening to both parent and child, the child psychiatrist most frequently suggests some environmental manipulation to ease the tension. An outpatient referral is made for a more extended evaluation beyond the scope of emergency consultation. Many of these aggressive children and parents carry diagnoses of depression and sociopathic or borderline character disorder. Some children also suffer from attention deficit disorders or conduct disorders. All of these problems may require long-term treatment.

In some cases, however, aggressive children and adolescents present a more serious and complicated picture in the emergency room. Some of these patients are angry, agitated, and out of control. Assessment of these children can be difficult and at times the consultant, especially the inexperienced consultant, may feel frightened or overwhelmed. It is important for the consultant to remember that the child is also frightened by his or her own loss of control and that the child is looking to the consultant as to a good parent, to help regain control in a nonthreatening, nonhumiliating way. The "uncontrollable" child should be interviewed in a quiet room in the emergency area. If it seems likely that the child will continue to act up, the evaluator should make certain that other staff members are readily available to help contain the child. The consultant must attempt in a calm, yet authoritative way to evaluate the situation.

The consultant has as one goal to determine whether this behavior is an exacerbation of a chronic pattern for this child, or whether this is a change in behavior reflecting a psychiatric condition, physical illness, or intoxication. Whatever the etiology of the behavior, the clinician's second goal is to understand the patient's problem and to assure the safety of the patient and others until longer-term treatment can be undertaken.

The psychiatric consultant must ascertain the following:

- Is there something specific that has triggered the patient's upset or outburst; is that behavior the culmination of a build-up of tension or did this behavior develop de novo?
- Is the patient's anger focused at someone or something in particular or is the aggression poorly organized and undirected?
- Does the child know what would help to make him or her feel better? Is this reasonable and is this possible?
- Has this child caused self-harm or harm to others or is he or she likely to do so?
- Does this child's reality-testing appear intact?

If the child has had acute change in behavior, organic causes should be considered before a psychiatric diagnosis can be made. Specifically, one should consider a neurologic problem such as a temporal lope epilepsy or organic brain syndrome secondary to infectious, metabolic, or oncologic process or intoxication. In terms of psychiatric diagnosis, one should consider hypomania, borderline personality with psychotic decompensation, and schizophrenia.

The consultant must keep in mind that patients with intoxication, organic brain syndrome, or acute psychosis are at particular risk for serious acting out of their aggressive feelings because of their poor impulse control, impaired reality-testing, and inadequate judgment.

Management should be aimed at treating the underlying disease. Although every effort should be made at resolving the situation verbally, at times the patient's behavior requires external controls. Before considering chemical intervention, it must be clear that this is not medically contraindicated. If this is the case, the patient must be physically restrained under observation until the agitation subsides or until medication can be used. Whenever medication is used, it must first be clearly explained to the patient that he or she is going to be given something that will help control aggression and help the patient to feel better.

For the moderately agitated and aggressive younger child who is not psychotic, diphenhydramine or hydroxyzine may be useful in reducing the disruptive behavior. Recommended dosage is 25 to 50 mg orally every 2 hours or until the behavior is diminished or the child is sedated. For acute treatment of children or adolescents with severe agitation or psychotic rage, major tranquilizers are recommended. The dosage regimen is similar to that detailed in the section in this chapter on psychosis.

Medication should be offered first in the oral form; if this is refused, in the injectable form. If it is given intramuscularly, the dose should be reduced by approximately one-half.

For the child with a psychiatric or medical illness precipitating aggressive behavior, inpatient evaluation is generally recommended. Placement in a facility that can provide a secure environment with 24-hour observation and protection is obviously recommended.

For the child or adolescent who does not have a primary psychiatric or medical illness, but who presents with aggressive behavior, the question for the psychiatric consultant becomes one primarily of safety for the patient and others. If chemical or physical restraints are necessary to control the patient, then a protective milieu may be necessary on a short-term basis.

HOMICIDE

Although it is relatively uncommon, some children, like adults, threaten and go on to commit serious acts of violence, including homicide. Young children and preadolescents who murder comprise a heterogeneous group that includes: normal children who kill in the course of play; those who mean only to hurt the victim; those who wish to kill out of anger, frustration, and hopelessness; those who act out what they have been taught; those who act out the unconscious wishes of others, particularly adults in their lives; and those children with severe developmental delays and organic, borderline, or psychotic disorders. (6).

Adolescents constitute the majority of homicidal youngsters. A substantial number of those who murder do so intentionally, their victims generally being family members or others well-known to them (7, 8). Malmquist (8) suggests that often the murderer and victim are involved in a sadomasochistic relationship through which the future perpetrator derives self-esteem. A threatened loss of this relationship is the precipitant to the homicidal ideation and act.

A significant number of these youngsters give clues prior to committing the act. Psychological autopsy reveals many premonitory signs (8):

- An object loss in an intense sadomasochistic relationship, as previously described, especially loss or perceived loss of a mother's love.
- A threat to one's sexuality or a homosexual threat.

- An ensuing shift in mood to hopelessness and often to self-hate.
- An increasing restlessness, agitation, and irritability.
- A use of drugs to alter feelings and impulses concomitantly impairing thought processes and diminishing ego controls.
- Increased somatization, hypochondriasis, or recurrent medical problems.
- A cry for help that may range from a muted call, often not perceived by others, to an explicit verbal warning or direct threat.
- An emotional crescendo with a loosening of thought processes and a breakdown of ego control over affective discharge.

Malmquist (8) suggests that, for homicidal individuals, in the face of hopelessness, helplessness, and ego disintegration, aggression is diverted away from the self (suicidal ideation) and projected onto the victim (homicidal ideation) in an attempt at survival.

While many individuals threaten "to kill," few seriously consider murder, and still fewer go on to commit murder. Although clear guidelines are not available for identifying those who will go on to kill, studies of adolescents who have murdered *do* indicate a particular high-risk population. This includes children or adolescents with: neurological impairment, schizophrenia, low IQ, history of school or work failure, unfavorable home situation (including early separation from parents and parental neglect or abuse), personal experience with brutality or violent death, history of fire-setting or cruelty to animals, and a history of other conduct disordered behavior, particularly in "loners." Those individuals with labile affect, prone to high anxiety, oriented toward action, and able to see killing as a feasible act are at particularly high risk. This risk is further raised in those who carry a psychiatric diagnosis, those who possess a weapon, those who have a plan of action, those whose anxiety and anger do not diminish during the course of psychiatric evaluation, and those who have previously killed (7, 9–11).

When an individual presents in the emergency room with

homicidal ideation, the psychiatric consultant must consider all of the aforementioned variables. It is, however, difficult for even the experienced clinician to predict, with accuracy, which individuals will go on to act on their homicidal threats. If there is *any* concern in the consultant's mind that there is serious risk of violence if the patient is released from the emergency room, a protective milieu must be considered. Many patients are relieved to be offered such treatment. In the case of the patient who refuses voluntary treatment, the consultant must be familiar with local laws for involuntary hospitalization.

CHILD ABUSE

Although child abuse has existed through the centuries, it is only within the last 25 years that this problem has begun to receive the attention it deserves. Statistics vary greatly concerning the number of children actually abused; a realistic estimation seems to be that well over 1,000,000 children are abused each year and of these, about 2,000 are killed (12). The child psychiatric consultant is generally involved with these children as they present in the emergency ward for medical treatment. In cases of flagrant abuse, the consultant may be called after the diagnosis has been made. In cases of more subtle abuse, the child psychiatric consultant may be asked for help in establishing the diagnosis.

Although child abuse includes physical abuse and neglect, sexual abuse and neglect, and emotional abuse and neglect, this section will deal primarily with physical abuse. Emergency treatment of sexual abuse is dealt with in the next chapter.

Physical abuse implies a nonaccidental injury to the child. Many families practice physical punishment, and there is wide cross-cultural variation in forms of such punishment. When this punishment results in an injury that requires medical attention, there is serious cause for concern. All states now have laws requiring that a physician who suspects physical abuse must report it to the appropriate authorities.

The first steps in detecting physical abuse are to recognize that it is a widespread phenomenon and to maintain a high level of suspicion when a child presents with an injury that cannot be explained by the parents to the satisfaction of the physician. Frequently, abusive parents alter their story as they tell it to different physicians or independently give differing histories of the injury, give explanations of the injury that are beyond the developmental capacity of the child, or place blame on the "babysitter." Less than 10 percent of abused children are abused by someone other than their parents or guardians (12). Any history or physical evidence of previous injuries and a delay in seeking medical attention should also raise questions.

Additionally, certain types of injuries are suggestive of abuse:

- Multiple injuries at various stages of resolution
- Bruises in the pattern of fingermarks or strap marks
- Burns from cigarette butts
- Scalding injuries
- Bite marks
- Bald spots (from hair pulling)
- Injuries of the long bones, especially dislocated metaphases or epiphyses, spiral fractures, or subperiosteal thickening
- Rupture of viscera

If abuse is suspected when the psychiatric consultant evaluates the child and parents, the consultant must remember that in most cases parents do not willfully intend to harm their children; rather, under stress, they have experienced a failure in their capacity to cope. Abusive parents are likely to be immature, with unmet dependency needs of their own. Most have come from unnurturing, unsupportive families. Many have themselves been abused. Most have poor impulse control.

In many cases the abused child is one who either poses a problem for the parent or places a demand on him or her. Infants and preschool children, nonverbal but demanding, are in the group statistically most likely to be abused. Also at high risk are children with medical problems and children who are mentally retarded, physically handicapped, neurologically impaired, hyperactive, colicky, or difficult to care for. A child to whom the parent has not bonded well is at particular risk.

The diagnosis of abuse depends heavily on a careful history, physical examination, x-ray and laboratory studies, and interview with the parents and child. Ideally, the history of the injury should be obtained separately from the child and the parents. For the most part, young children do not fabricate physical abuse. *Any allegations they make should be taken seriously.*

Physical examination should be directed not only to the presenting injury, but also to the possibility of old injuries. A bone survey is useful in providing additional data. For the child reported to be "an easy bruiser," a coagulation profile may be in order.

The results of history and physical examination should be carefully documented.

A joint interview with the parents and child provides additional data. It is important to assess the child's relationship with the parent. Does the child seem frightened? Does the parent seem to have unreasonable expectations of the child? Does the child have the role of parentified child, caring for the parent and for siblings? If these questions can be answered in the affirmative, then the suspicion increases that abuse has occurred. The final diagnosis of abuse is usually a joint decision involving pediatrician, child psychiatrist, social worker, and a legal consultant. In many hospitals all suspected abuse cases are reviewed by an advocate group and a team determination made.

It is generally advised that a child with suspected abuse be hospitalized. Hospitalization allows both for treatment of injury and protection of the child. In some instances the child may be allowed to return home. Such a decision is based on the judgment that the child will be safe. If this is at all in question, the child *must* be hospitalized.

In all cases of suspected child abuse it is mandatory that the physician file a report with the protective service agencies.

It is also the physician's responsibility to inform the parents of the diagnosis that has been made. The medical reasons for the diagnosis and the legal requirement to report such cases should be explained. Discussion with the parent should be nonjudgmental. Parents should be told what will happen following the receipt of the report, including subsequent investigation by a social service worker. The clinician should emphasize that reporting of the incident will enable them to receive helpful services. Many parents feel relieved and supported by these approaches. Others appear angry and indignant. Considerable skill may be required on the part of the physician to help parents accept what is being done is out of concern for a child and for them. A physician who can communicate concern for a child and family can do much to pave the way for successful intervention.

PSYCHOSIS

Psychosis is relatively uncommon in childhood and adolescence. When it does occur, the psychiatric consultant must determine the etiology of the condition. The major emergency considerations are the differential diagnosis of functional and organic psychoses in relation to the risk of suicidal or homicidal behaviors.

Functional psychosis is less common in children than adults and is more difficult to diagnose in childhood because it may be less obvious to the untrained observer. While mid- and older adolescents may present with symptoms similar to those of schizophrenic or manic-depressive adults, children and young adolescents characteristically present with a history of gradual deterioration. They often have evidence of progressive social withdrawal, emotional blunting, and a decline in school performance. Their odd behavior has typically been ongoing and is frequently seen by their parents more as a part of their character and less as a part of a psychiatric disorder. When schizophrenia does occur in childhood, it is more often an undifferentiated type than paranoid or catatonic, although older adolescents may have these latter subtypes.

When these children come to the attention of the emergency room psychiatrist, they often present not with a picture of acute schizophrenic decompensation, but with such symptoms as suicidal ideation or behavior, increased agitation and aggression, or extreme anxiety. By focusing both on mental status examination and on history, a tentative diagnosis can be made and an appropriate treatment undertaken. Children with acute psychotic decompensation are often a danger to themselves or others and often need emergency treatment in a hospital setting.

In children with "quiet psychoses," extreme stress may potentiate an acute psychotic decompensation. In these instances, the child may exhibit the more characteristic signs of psychosis such as hallucinations, delusions, or frankly bizarre behavior.

Children with organic psychoses typically present with an acute picture. Their decompensation is usually of recent onset and there is no history of a precipitating emotional stress. They are often agitated, disorganized, and disoriented. Their memory may be impaired. They may be experiencing hallucinations. Frequently, these hallucinations are visual rather than more characteristic auditory hallucinations of schizophrenia (an exception being the auditory hallucinations seen in alcoholic hallucinosis).

Many medical conditions may be associated with acute psychosis. These included neurologic, infectious, metabolic, oncologic, and immunologic processes. In addition, acute psychosis can be associated with alcohol or drug intoxication or withdrawal, and with vitamin deficiency.

Neurological disorders are among the most common causes of organic psychosis. Meningitis, encephalitis, cerebral vascular accidents, subarachnoid hemorrhages, and subdural hematoma can be associated with acute behavioral changes presenting as acute psychosis. Children with congenital heart disease and leukemia are at special risk for cerebral vascular complications and their neurological status should be evaluated before their behavioral changes can be attributed to stress from their illness.

Patients with brain tumors occasionally present with symptoms of acute psychosis. Metastases to the central nervous system (CNS) may also present a psychotic picture. Children with seizure disorders may present with interictal or postictal behavior that can be mistaken for psychotic behavior. Symptoms resembling childhood schizophrenia may be seen in children with early neurodegenerative disease.

Patients with metabolic disorders, especially myxedema, thyrotoxicosis, or Cushing's disease (and less frequently diabetes) may appear to have acute psychosis. Similarly, patients with pulmonary disease resulting in anoxia may also present with psychotic-like symptoms. In these patients, the obvious physical signs and symptoms will suggest organic etiology. Diagnoses can then be confirmed by appropriate laboratory tests.

Porphyria and Wilson's disease may present with psychiatric manifestations before other evidence of the disease is present. Patients with lupus erythematous can develop symptoms of organic psychosis. Sometimes it is difficult to know if the disease or the treatment for the disease (steroids) is the cause of the psychiatric symptomatology.

Deficiency of nicotinic acid or thiamine may cause symptoms of psychosis. Intoxication with lead may do the same.

Some medications produce CNS side effects that resemble psychotic-like symptoms. Anticholinergic agents, such as those found in over-the-counter sleep-inducing preparations, as well as antihistaminic agents are known in toxic amounts to produce psychosis. Overdosage of sedative hypnotics or abrupt withdrawal of these agents may also result in a psychotic state. A careful drug history is essential for accurate diagnosis and management.

Intoxication with street drugs is particularly problematic in that it may be unclear if the acute psychotic symptomatology is a direct result of the drug use or if the drug has precipitated psychosis in a predisposed individual. Psychoses induced by LSD or psilocybin (PCP) may mimic acute schizophrenic decompensation. Amphetamine-induced psychosis can mimic a manic episode or paranoid schizophrenia. LSD, PCP, and amphetamine-induced psychoses (in long-time users) can persist for weeks to months after the drugs have been cleared from the system. LSD and PCP are also associated with flashbacks, which may include hallucinations or distortions of thought.

Patients who abuse drugs are frequently unable to give an accurate history of what they have taken. Many street drugs are impure or mixed with other drugs unknown to the patient. It is important to be familiar with the physical signs and symptoms associated with intoxication with the various hallucinogenic drugs. Such familiarity helps the consultant in making a working drug diagnosis in the absence of an accurate history and lab data.

A toxic screen may be helpful in determining what drug has been taken. It is important for the consultant to be familiar with the substances that are routinely included in a hospital's toxic screen. If the consultant suspects intoxication with a drug for which routine screening is not done, the consultant may request that the laboratory look specifically for that drug. Certain drugs leave the bloodstream so rapidly that they may be undetectable in a serum toxic screen. For this reason, both urine and serum screen should be sent to the laboratory. Since there appears to be a high percentage of false negative reports from routine screening, the consultant is best advised to rely heavily on history, physical findings, and mental status examination and to use the laboratory results as diagnostic only if they confirm the suspicions (Table 1) (13,14).

Once the safety of the patient has been established and the etiology of the psychosis has been determined, treatment decisions must be made. The acute treatment of functional psychosis depends on the presentation of the patient. If the child presents with a major change in personality or behavior, if the child is extremely distressed or anxious, or if the child is hallucinating, delusional, suicidal, or overly aggressive, hospitalization is the initial treatment of choice. In the hospital, the child must be maintained in a safe, structured, nonstimulating environment with close observation. Visitors should be restricted. Nursing care should be delivered by a core group of nurses. Reassurance, support, and consistency are the most important therapeutic maneuvers.

For the severely disturbed child, psychopharmacologic agents

Table 1. Signs and Symptoms of Substance Abuse

Substance	Psychiatric Symptoms Following Intoxication	Physical Signs Following Intoxication
Amphetamines	Talkativeness, restlessness, anxiety, agitation, elation, visual and tactile hallucinations, paranoid ideation. Psychosis that can occur from days to months following ingestion in those who have been moderate to large drug abusers over long periods of time. Symptoms similar to those of functional psychosis, not intoxication.	Dilated pupils (responsive to light), tachycardia, diaphoresis, tremulousness, hyperreflexia, stereotyped movement. If severe: hypertension, hyperpyrexia, cardiac arrhythmia.
Cocaine	Similar to amphetamine intoxication but much shorter duration.	Similar to amphetamine, but shorter duration.
LSD and mescaline	Apprehension, panic, perceptual distortion, including slowed sense of time and synesthesias, depersonalization, derealization, hallucinations (visual or auditory).	Same as above but less severe.
PCP (and ketamine)	Anxiety, euphoria, disorientation, hallucinations (suicidal behavior is not uncommon). May be associated with waxing and waning of psychiatric symptoms for up to 1 week.	Pupils normal or small, nystagmus (vertical or horizontal), muscular rigidity, grimacing, numbness or decreased sensory perception, hypertension.

may be necessary. Major tranquilizers are the treatment of choice. Chlorpromazine is approved for children 6 months and older, thioridazine for children 3 years and older, and haloperidol for children 8 years and older. Table 2 details use of these drugs for emergency treatment of acute psychosis. These doses should be adjusted accordingly for children under age 6 (15). (See also Chapter 9.) In the case of organic psychoses, definitive treatment should be directed at the underlying disease. Acute management of the psychotic episode is similar to the management of such an episode in patients with functional psychosis. If agitation is severe, psychotropic intervention may be necessary, but this must be done with consideration of the underlying disease process.

In the instance of drug-induced psychoses, if the patient does know specifically what has been taken, management decisions may be simplified.

For patients who are intoxicated with anticholinergic or antihistaminic drugs, physostigmine provides specific and rapid relief of symptoms. Major tranquilizers are specifically contraindicated. Use of them exacerbates symptomatology (13).

In the case of cocaine-induced psychotic reactions, the psychosis is generally of such short duration that medication is

Table 2. Drugs Used for Emergency Treatment of Acute Psychosis

Drug	Initial Dose	Sequential Dosage
Chlorpromazine (oral)	0.5–1.0 mg/kg	0.5–2.0 mg/kg q 2h–4h until child responds or until side effects contraindicate, up to about 4 doses.
Thioridazine	0.5–1.0 mg/kg	Same as chlorpromazine.
Haloperidol	0.5 mg (total dose)	0.01–0.1 mg/kg q 2h–4h until responsive or side effects are limiting, up to about 4 doses.

not necessary. If medication is required, use of a major tranquilizer is recommended.

For amphetamine intoxication, management includes:

- Increasing amphetamine excretion by acidification of the urine with oral ammonium chloride
- Producing adrenergic blockage in the CNS by use of a major tranquilizer, preferably chlorpromazine or haloperidol
- Propranolol is also useful in blocking the amphetamine-induced β adrenergic hyperactivity (13).

In the case of hallucinogen-induced psychosis, there is no specific treatment. Reassurance is the most important therapeutic measure (13).

When it is not known what medication the patient has ingested, sedation and tranquilization should be attempted only if the patient's agitation or anxiety is quite severe and other measures of management have failed.

If medication is necessary, benzodiazepines are the drugs of choice; they provide sedation with a minimum of other undesired side effects. Major tranquilizers and barbiturates are particularly risky when the pharmacology of the underlying intoxication is not known. In patients with anticholinergic intoxication, phenothiazines may precipitate agitation, delirium, and a drop in blood pressure. In patients who have abused PCP, phenothiazines may cause an alpha blockage precipitating life-threatening postural hypotension. Barbiturates can produce depressed respiration and coma. If a major tranquilizer must be used, the smallest possible amount of high potency drug, such as haloperidol, is recommended. In all instances, the patient must be carefully monitored.

EATING DISORDERS

Patients with eating disorders may present as psychiatric emergencies. Since morbidity and mortality rates in these patients are among the highest for psychiatric disorders, it is essential that the psychiatrist in the emergency room be familiar with signs and symptoms of these disorders and with indications for hospitalization. Further, the risk of suicide in this population is increased.

It is estimated that serious eating disorders affect 5 to 10 percent of teenage girls and young women (16). Although males may also suffer from these disorders, over 90 percent of anorexics and bulimics are women. These disorders most often begin in teenage years. Both usually begin with a moderate effort to lose weight that escalates to a relentless attempt to achieve thinness. Restrictive anorexia is characterized by a severe reduction in caloric intake. There is a refusal to maintain normal body weight, a loss of more than 25 percent of original body weight, a disturbance of body image, and an intense fear of becoming fat. Bulimic anorexia nervosa is characterized by a restriction of caloric intake alternating with episodes of binge eating, usually followed by self-induced vomiting or use of laxatives or diuretics. Both syndromes affect multiple organ systems and both can be fatal.

In the case of the restrictive anorexic, the physical complications of concern to the emergency room psychiatrist are, for the most part, those of starvation. These include the inability to maintain body temperature, dehydration, total body sodium and potassium loss, and cardiac arrhythmia due to either electrolyte imbalance or anatomical cardiac changes secondary to starvation.

For the bulimic anorexic, physical complications are associated with binging and purging and include the risks of acute gastric dilatation and rupture, Mallory-Weiss tear, aspiration, and electrolyte disturbance. Diuretic abuse, cathartic abuse, and self-induced vomiting all predispose to serious hypokalemia, which can precipite fatal arrhythmia. Ipecac abuse can cause direct myocardial dysfunction and precipitate sudden death.

The physician in the emergency room must assess the physical and emotional status of the patient and the risk for death. Indications for hospitalization include:

- history of a recent precipitous drop in weight or history of a steady drop in weight over the last several months ap-

proaching loss of 25 to 30 percent of body weight
- history of increased binging or vomiting or increased use of cathartics or diuretics to a frequency or intensity that seem life-endangering
- history of change in mental status with increasing depression or suicidality or emerging psychotic decompensation
- metabolic disturbance such as serious alteration in vital signs, imbalance of electrolytes (especially low sodium or potassium), elevation of blood urea nitrogen with otherwise normal renal function
- history of chest pain or arrhythmia or presence of an abnormal EKG

Initials treatment should address the medical or psychiatric indications precipitating the hospitalization. Further treatment should include continued medical management, individual and family psychotherapy, and behavioral treatment for restitution of weight and control of binging and purging. Psychopharmacologic intervention may be useful.

School Refusal ("School Phobias")

Although not an emergency as described elsewhere in this chapter, and although rarely a presenting complaint in the emergency room, the school-refusing child or adolescent requires rapid assessment and intervention in many instances (17). In this respect some child psychiatrists consider school refusal an emergency. The danger or risk in this syndrome is the possibility of the child developing entrenched avoidance of school. When this occurs there is more likelihood of chronic developmental interference taking place in a system that can be increasingly rigid and therapeutically difficult to move. Thus, whether primary as cause of referral, or secondary but discovered in the course of diagnostic assessments in any setting, the recognition of this problem requires several subsequent steps:

- The initial task is to complete the standard work-up with

particular attention to the time of onset of the school avoidance and any possible precipitants.
- Separation difficulties, most usually between the mother and index patient, are omnipresent. Family issues such as losses and marital stress should be explored.
- Prior history of separation anxiety disorders or panic disorders in the parents is useful to document because these conditions may indicate responsiveness to pharmacologic intervention (see below).
- Underlying psychiatric illness should be carefully searched out. In younger children (pre-pubertal), fixed and serious psychopathology is less likely to coexist with school refusal. However, in pubertal children or adolescents, school avoidance is more likely to be associated with major psychiatric illness, including the schizoid disorders and schizophrenia.

When satisfied that no other underlying conditions require prior treatment, the management of school refusal is based on the child psychiatrist facilitating mutual mastery of the underlying and sometimes *unconscious* separation anxiety in child and parent(s). Principles of management include:

- The establishment of firm authoritative control in the hands of one person, usually the child psychiatrist.
- Reassurance of both child and parent(s) that, despite the anxiety of the child, both parties will be "all right" apart and that the child must be in school.
- Implementation of a structured plan involving the specific reality details of the morning departure for school, attempting to foresee all possible scenarios; this may require the collaboration of school personnel such as principals, teachers, or a favorite nurse who can unwittingly undermine the child's return to school.
- The use of tricyclic antidepressants, which may be in order as an aid to reducing the child's anxiety (see Chapter 9).

When given an adequate trial of 5 to 10 school days, such a plan's efficacy is useful diagnostically. The reasonably healthy child and family will be able, with support, to resolve school refusal. Psychotherapy of the etiologic issues can then begin. However, when such an approach cannot be implemented or fails, one is generally forced to deal with more serious psychiatric illness.

REFERENCES

1. Khan AU: Psychiatric Emergencies in Pediatrics. Chicago, Year Book Medical Publications, 1979

2. Pfeffer CR: Suicidal behavior of children: a review with implications for research and practice. Am J Psychiatry 138:154–159, 1981

3. Pfeffer CR, Conte HR, Plutchik R, et al: Suicidal behavior in latency age children. J Amer Acad Child Psychiatry 19:703–710, 1980

4. Myerson AT, Glick RA, Kier A: Suicide, in Psychiatric Emergencies. Edited by Myerson AT, Robbins E, Talbott J. New York, Grune & Stratton, 1976

5. Pfeffer CR: Interventions for suicidal children and their parents. Suicide Life Threat Behav 12:240–245, 1982

6. Petti T: The juvenile murderer, in Child Psychiatry and the Law. Edited by Schetky D, Benedek E. New York, Brunner/Mazel, 1980

7. Sendi I, Blomgren P: A comparative study of the predictive criteria in the predisposition of homicidal adolescents. Am J Psychiatry 132:4, 1975

8. Malmquist C: Premonitory signs of homicidal aggression in juveniles. Am J Psychiatry 121:461–465, 1971

9. Bender L: Children and adolescents who have killed. Am J Psychiatry 116:510–513, 1959

10. Lewis DO, Shanok SS, Pincus JH, et al: Violent juvenile delinquents, psychiatric, neurological, psychological and abuse factors. Amer Acad Child Psychiatry 18:307–319, 1979

11. Allen NH: Homocide prevention and intervention. Suicide Life Threat Behav 11:167–179, 1981
12. McNeese MC, Hebeler JR: *CIBA Clinical Symposia*, Vol 29. Summit, NJ, CIBA Pharmaceutical Company, 1977
13. Greenblatt DJ, Shader RI: Bad trips, in Manual of Psychiatric Therapeutics. Edited by Shader RI. Boston, Little, Brown and Co, 1975, pp 185–193
14. *The Medical Letter*, September 5, 1980
15. Popper CW, Famularo R: Child and adolescent psychopharmacology, in Developmental-Behavioral Pediatrics. Edited by Levine MD, Carery WB, Crocker AC, et al. Philadelphia, WB Saunders Co, 1983, pp 1138–1159
16. Herzog DB, Copeland PM: Eating disorders. N Engl J Med 313:295–303, 1985
17. Halmi, KA: Anorexia nervosa, in Comprehensive Textbook of Psychiatry IV, Vol. 2. Edited by Kaplan HI, Sadock BJ. Baltimore, Williams & Wilkins Co, 1985, pp 1882–1891

Chapter 11

Emergencies II: Sexual Abuse and Rape in Childhood

Maria Sauzier, M.D.

Catherine Mitkus, LIC.S.W., M.S.W.

Sexual abuse and rape of children, increasingly common emergency room conditions, evoke powerful emotional reactions not only in trainees but in all professionals. Medicine and psychiatry have only very recently begun to face these issues, paralleling a societal development toward endowing children with more rights. This has led to complex debates about the interface between parental authority, the right to privacy within the family, and the protection of children (1). A second controversy relates to professional intervention, and who bears the primary responsibility: medicine, psychiatry, child protective social service agencies, the police, or district attorneys. Different states are using a variety of solutions to this problem, but most new legislation stresses the need for cooperation between professionals from mental health, protective services, and the judicial system (2).

The goal of this chapter is to give clinicians a basic framework of knowledge encompassing clinical terminology (sexual abuse, misuse, incest, rape) and related legal issues (mandated reporting, confidentiality). Clinical issues are reviewed following the format used in psychiatric diagnostic evaluations and treatment planning. The whole family is seen as the object of intervention. Child victims, perpetrators, and nonabusing mothers, fathers, and siblings are briefly described.

Intervention with and treatment of sexually abused children still present great challenges because they are new frontiers: treatment programs are at the most 10 to 15 years old. There are at present no long-term outcome studies comparing different intervention strategies. Nevertheless, contemporary clinicians agree that the child who presents with a history of sexual abuse or rape needs more than traditional psychiatric treatment (3). We thus speak of "intervention." This includes the following:

- Psychiatric evaluation and treatment,
- Child protective investigation, and
- Legal involvement.

These facets of intervention need to be described together, just as they need to be interwoven in clinical practice. For the child psychiatrist, treatment of a sexually abused child may offer a unique opportunity to cooperate with child protective and law enforcement systems under very stressful circumstances.

Sexual Abuse

Background

Information about sexual abuse comes from case histories (4, 5), small-scale psychologic studies (6, 7), or large-scale sociologic studies (8, 9). One broad psychologic research project has recently been conducted at New England Medical Center, using 181 cases of sexual abuse (156 confirmed, 25 unconfirmed) (10). Concomitant with data collection was the provision of therapy for the child and the child's family, including the offender. The children seen were between 6 months and 18 years old; 72 percent were girls. The sexual abuse reported ranged from exposure to intercourse, with some genital contact in 88 percent of the cases. Ninety-four percent of the offenders were male, ranging from teenage babysitters to grandfathers. Their average age was 29. Only 3 percent of offenders were total strangers. Incest in the biologic sense occurred in 41 percent of the cases seen. If one includes parental figures such as live-in boyfriends, the figure rises to 62 percent. Only 21 percent of abuse occurred as one single incident of rape or incest. Most occurred over a variable period of time, some spanning more than 5 years, with a frequency varying between several times for the whole span or years, to more than weekly. Most abuse incidents occurred in places familiar to the child, like the child's home or the perpetrator's home. The families studied were representative of the greater Boston population in terms of race, religion, and socioeconomic status. The only remarkable demographic difference found was a higher preponderance of households headed by single parents. Although this research is not described in detail here, it informs all aspects of this chapter (the research was supported by grant #80-JN-AX-0001 [S2] from the Office of Juvenile Justice and Delinquency Prevention).

Clinical Terminology

Sexual abuse, sexual misuse, incest, and rape of children have overlapping definitions. Nevertheless, it is important to spell out the differences and their implications. *Sexual abuse* covers the widest range of activities in which a child is used for the sexual gratification of an adult. By definition, a child cannot be a consenting partner to any sexual interaction with an adult. A child can also be abused by another child if the perpetrator is significantly older than the victim, or uses threats, intimidation, or force to create a power differential (e.g., as exists between a babysitter of any age and his or her charges).

Sexual misuse occurs when the adult is truly not aware of any sexual gratification he or she may be receiving (e.g., as when a parent continues to treat a genital or anal irritation with checking, washing, and ointment originally prescribed but no longer necessary). *Incest* in the strict sense occurs when blood relatives interact sexually. The broader and more current definition includes relatives who are not consanguineous (e.g, an uncle by marriage), as well as stepparents, live-in partners of parents, or any adult who is given parental authority in the household. *Rape* implies the more overt use of violence and occurs more often in isolated incidents. This contrasts with the usually progressive nature of sexual abuse, where there is a continuum of sexual interactions (e.g., cuddling, which can lead to fondling, which can lead to penetration). Sexual abuse or rape do not imply anything about the kinds of sexual acts performed, although in the legal definition rape involves some penetration of a body orifice. Rape is more often perpetrated by a stranger, sexual abuse by a person known to the child. Both may be incestuous or not.

Sexual abuse and, in particular, incest may thus be complicated by the fact that the child has a relationship with the offender that encompasses more than just the abuse. Incest strongly implies individual and family dynamics allowing or even prompting it to occur. There are, thus, certain common features found in incest families that require therapeutic intervention.

In the sections that follow, sexual abuse and incest will be discussed concurrently, followed by a discussion of specific issues concerning rape.

Legal Issues

The last several years have seen a dramatic and steady increase of reported cases of sexual abuse of children. In Massachusetts, 1,400 cases of sexual abuse were reported in 1981, 2,142 in 1982, and 5,065 in 1984 (11). This increase in reports is seen by most experts as due to stronger mandated reporting laws, media attention to the problem, and more sophisticated and reliable responses from child protective services. Child psychiatrists should be aware of the legal requirements in their state. In Massachusetts, for example, professionals including physicians, nurses, therapists, and teachers are mandated to report findings or suspicions of abuse to the Department of

Social Services; false allegations made in good faith cannot be held against the reporter.

Issues of confidentiality may arise when a child reveals sexual abuse in ongoing therapy, leading to ethical and therapeutic dilemmas, although the mandated reporting of information regarding child abuse is exempt from the privilege of confidentiality. In accordance with the literature, reporting is strongly recommended (3). The incest family in particular is riddled with secrets that empower the abuser at the expense of other family members. The therapist who participates in the secret thus loses effectiveness in the eyes of the child and of the offender. In addition, many offenders actually want to be stopped by outside intervention. Even more difficult are those situations in which a child gives clues but does not openly talk about being abused.

Mandated reporting of serious cases to the District Attorney is a recent development in several states (e.g., Massachusetts), but does not imply automatic prosecution. It does, however, have implications for the format of clinical interviews and medical records, as discussed later. Parameters of confidentiality privileges vary across disciplines and should be reviewed accordingly.

CLINICAL ISSUES IN SEXUAL ABUSE

Presenting Complaint

Sexual abuse will only be considered in a differential diagnosis if one's consciousness has been raised to such problems. Minimization of the problem of sexual abuse of children is related not only to the wish to deny its existence, but also to the paucity of clear clinical indicators.

Unfortunately for diagnostic purposes, with the exceptions of medical signs, the various symptoms seen are not in themselves indicative of sexual abuse but are nonspecific and related to the developmental stage of the child. For the most part, sexual abuse of children does not require the use of overt violence; children can be made to comply with the use of authority, bribes, or misrepresentation of social values alone. Thus only rarely are there bruises and cuts to alert the clinician. Nevertheless, there are some presentations that should always lead to an investigation:

- A child who states that he or she has been sexually abused has to be taken seriously and the allegations investigated. In the New England Medical Center research, only five families presented with children who made false allegations (of a total of 181 cases) (10).
- A parent who states that his or her child has been sexually abused also has to be taken seriously. This is particularly important when the child is preverbal. It is extremely complex, however, when the accusing parent and the alleged offender are battling over custody or visitation.

Physical Signs and Symptoms

- Genital or anal tears, bruises or irritations, discharge, and sexually transmitted disease, although rare, are the most specific indicators.
- Encopresis can be associated with anal rape.
- Enuresis may be a symptom of regression, overexcitation, or fears related to sexual abuse.
- Psychosomatic symptoms, such as headaches or stomachaches, may be present.

Emotional and Behavior Symptoms

- Nightmares or night terrors may follow abuse.
- Clinginess, whininess, or refusal to stay with a specific person (e.g., a particular babysitter or uncle) may indicate abuse by that person.
- Preschool children may exhibit hypersexual or deviant behavior, such as excessive public masturbation, show-and-tell or doctor games played in a driven or overanxious way, and especially abuse of another child. These may be expressions or reenactments of sexual overstimulation or abuse and require investigation.

- Older children, particularly teenagers, may present acting out symptoms, including truancy, lying, stealing, promiscuity, alcohol abuse, suicide attempts, and running away from home. Many runaways and prostitutes have a history of sexual abuse.

All of these symptoms are nonspecific, can be multidetermined, and can express different kinds of distress. Some children, particularly latency age children, may exhibit no symptoms at all and may be abused for years, until adolescence, without divulging the secret.

Revelation of Abuse

The revelation of sexual abuse may be purposeful or accidental. Purposeful disclosure is usually made to a parent or another trusted adult. Accidental disclosure is not overtly wanted by anyone, not even the victim, and may follow physical findings (e.g., sexually transmitted disease, pregnancy) or observation of the abuse or its consequences by someone who then reveals it.

Revelation during psychotherapy may be purposeful, accidental, or both. Clues given may be drawings (e.g., genitalia), hypersexual behavior (e.g., seductive or excessive masturbatory activity in the therapeutic sessions), or veiled references to secret pacts, excluding siblings and mother. In the past these clues were usually understood to relate to fantasy material and wishes. Today we know that sexual abuse occurs widely. The task of the clinician in such a situation is a difficult one: to elicit further information without leading the child to feel more stimulated, intruded on, or even revictimized.

Disclosure of sexual abuse *always* precipitates a *crisis* situation for the victim and the victim's family. For the victim, revelation offers hope for change, but also fear of the consequences. In cases of incest, the victim has kept the secret to prevent being blamed, shamed, or losing the affection of the offender. For the non-offending parent, usually the mother, the crisis is severe and may impede her ability to make choices that protect and support the victim. For the offender, the first response to the revelation is usually denial, with or without attempts to lead the victim to retract.

CRISIS INTERVENTION

Key Issues in Crisis Management of Sexual Abuse and Incest Cases

The entire family is in a complicated state of crisis. For each member, the timing and intensity varies. The revelation and its impact are seen in a different light by each member. The clinician's role is diverse, comprehensive, and flexible, going beyond the classic model of the neutral, insight-oriented therapist. Teamwork is *essential*. Extensive advocacy, collaboration, and liaison work with courts, the Department of Social Services (DSS), and other providers may be necessary.

Chief Sources of Distress and Fears for Children and Siblings

- Fears of family destruction or abandonment.
- Fears of vulnerability to future harm (for siblings: "Will I be next in line?").
- Sense of shame and devaluation.
- Fears of punishment, reprisal, rejection from parents.
- Guilt (participation in something "bad"; "survivor guilt"; "failed rescue attempts"; guilt for experience of physical pleasure).
- Disappointment and sense of betrayal from parenting figures.
- Stress due to knowledge of incest and pressure to maintain secrecy.
- Stress related to premature stimulation of sexual drives.
- Stress related to change in family dynamics (possibly structures) to new and unknown modes of functioning.

In non-incest cases stress is related to fears and helplessness vis-à-vis the outside perpetrator who may still be in the neighborhood.

Chief Sources of Distress for Mothers

- Pressure to make immediate decisions when capacities to think clearly are highly compromised by the shock of the revelation.
- Fears of family disruption, legal proceedings and criminal prosecution, financial crises, and public exposure.
- Confused notions regarding whom to believe, implications of allegations, impact on each member.
- Confusing, stressful, and complicated interactions with a variety of systems and people at a point of crisis (e.g., police, DSS, medical providers, psychiatric professionals, courts).
- Enormous uncertainty and sudden loss of control.

Chief Sources of Distress for Incestuous Fathers

- Fears of prosecution.
- Humiliation and shame.
- Fears of family abandonment, rejection, disruption.
- Confused notions regarding source of responsibility, impact on the child, clinical and legal implications.

Initial Interventions

The response to a sexually abused child requires *action*. For clinicians trained in the passive or expectant mode, this may present some difficulty.

The first question requiring clarification concerns the referral source. If child protective services are involved, they usually make the referral to the clinic; cooperation with them is mandatory as well as helpful. If a parent or other adult has referred the child, a decision to report the abuse, based on state regulations, needs to be made. The initial goals of the intervention are as follows:

- Find out what has happened from the child.

- Assess the acute safety of the child and clinical diagnostic profile.
- Assess mother's ability to protect.
- Assess father's ability to cease his behavior and obtain help.
- Formulate initial findings, diagnostic impressions, and *initial* disposition plans.
- Help family members deal with their reactions to the stress precipitated by the revelation.
- If non-incest: assess family's safety in the neighborhood.

Stated briefly, there are several essential steps to be taken after the revelation of sexual abuse:

- *Interview of the child* alone is essential for diagnostic purposes, to elicit the information necessary to plan for the child's safety, and to begin the treatment process by supporting the child's strengths that led to the disclosure of the abuse.
- *Interview of the nonabusing parent* provides support and nonjudgmental suggestions about how to help the abused child. Fostering the highest level of functioning, despite the crisis of revelation, takes precedence over exploratory work at this point in time. Information regarding the parent's ability to protect the child from further harm should be gathered.
- *Interview of the offender*, an essential component of the evaluation of an incestuous family, provides information about the family dynamics and the child's safety. The offender may react to the disclosure with serious psychopathology, including suicidal or homicidal impulses and actions. In a non-incest abuse situation, access to the offender may be limited but should always be sought.
- *Interview of siblings* may reveal other victims, or may elicit reactions that can be detrimental to the victimized child (e.g., blaming the victim for the act).
- A *referral for a physical examination*, either to the family pediatrician or to one familiar with and sensitive to the issues of sexually abused children, should be made. The physical examination may detect consequences of the abuse

that require treatment (e.g., sexually transmitted disease, pregnancy) or that may be important elements in case of prosecution of the offender. The examination should always respond to the child's and parent's spoken and unspoken fears (e.g., "Is the child physically marred for life?").

- *Cooperation* with child protective and legal services elicits their help and informs them of clinical needs and issues. Their work as investigators and case administrators is essential and leaves the clinician more freedom to maintain supportive and psychotherapeutic roles.
- *Assessment of the child's safety* is the primary consideration. Many factors are relevant, including:

  - The identity of the *offender*, the access he has to the child, his modus operandi (e.g., using violence or not), his acknowledgment or denial of the abuse.
  - The age and the stage of development of the *child*, the child's strengths (e.g., a trusting relationship with mother, the therapist, or other adults; an ability to say no), weaknesses (e.g., mental retardation, any other impairment, ambivalence toward the nonabusing parent, need to side with the offender).
  - The response of the *mother*, whether she can side with the child without blame or punishment, whether she is appropriately angry with the offender, whether she can place the child's needs over her own attachment to the offender, and her own needs.
  - The response of *siblings*, their situation in the family (are they at risk?), their response toward the victim (e.g., blaming the victim and siding with the offender, thus increasing the mother's dilemma of choosing between them).

- A *separation* between the child and the alleged offender is always indicated. In cases of incest, the offending adult should leave the household, at least temporarily, thus acknowledging that the offender accepts the blame. Financial responsibilities, however, should continue to be met. Removing the victimized child from the home should be seen as the last resort in families that cannot protect the victim from further harm.

Interviewing Technique

The passive observing and evaluating approach forms only the initial baseline for assessing a sexually abused child. Getting acquainted, forming an alliance, getting a sense of the child's life and areas of strengths and weakness, and performing a mental status examination are all important features of the assessment; they may not lead, however, to any discussion of the sexual abuse. Concrete and direct questioning about the alleged abuse is usually the best approach, with attention to verbal and nonverbal reactions, just as in any child therapy setting. Anatomically correct dolls can be invaluable in eliciting information, especially from the preverbal or reticent child. The victim needs to be reassured about the positive value of telling the secret, and also told that the child's parents need to know and that this may lead to other people trying to help the whole family. At the same time, the clinician needs to be aware of trying not to ask leading questions. The child usually experiences relief coupled with great fear of family disintegration or retaliation. False reassurances about the immediate consequences (e.g., "I'm sure your Daddy will be able to stay with you") can only lead to disappointment and a breach of trust. A child can usually understand that the family situation needs to change so that the child and the offender can both receive help. Interview each involved member *separately*. Family meetings are contraindicated at the point of revelation and often throughout the initial crisis period. Most children are unable to talk freely in front of their parents, fearing accusations of disloyalty, rejection, or punishment. Protection includes a safe place to talk, even for siblings.

Interviewing the Sexually Abused Child

Once the immediate crisis situation has been responded to, the child psychiatrist can turn to gathering more detailed clinical data. Sexual abuse of children usually occurs as an extension of an existing relationship between victim and offender. The clinician thus needs to unravel the history of the abuse, and of the ties between the three main protagonists: the victim, his or her nonoffending parent(s), and the offender. The possibilities are vast, particularly when the offender has a relationship based on power with both the child and the nonoffending parent. The outline described here can provide only guiding principles. Again, the clinician, beginner or not, is urged to keep an open mind in this new field. Incest, a more complex and more frequent situation, will be described in more detail.

Victims

Blaming the victim is a universal defense. It serves to reduce the anxiety aroused and to contain the fear that "this could happen to me or my child." The psychiatric literature has sometimes participated by describing sexually abused children as seductive, precocious, and beautiful, which was seen as making them responsible for seducing the adult (16). The error lies in a confusion of cause and effect; some sexually abused children are indeed seductive with their therapists, as well as with anyone else, because they have been taught that this behavior pleases and gets them the gratification they need.

More recent literature focuses on the wide range of presentations seen in sexually abused children (17). On average they show more psychopathology than children in control groups but less than those in a psychiatric clinic population (10). This confirms clinical observations that some sexually abused children show no signs of distress at revelation, whereas others show serious signs and symptoms. Self-esteem may be normal in younger children, particularly if the abuse was nonviolent and the response to the revelation was caring and supportive. They may not have yet perceived the pathologic nature of what has happened to them. It may only be later, sometimes as late as adolescence or adulthood, that they come to realize that they have been misled and abused by a trusted adult.

The absence of symptoms in an abused child, shortly after revelation, thus needs to be carefully evaluated. Children who are asymptomatic may not require more than short-term therapy or crisis intervention and case management to secure their safety. Long-term therapy may or may not become necessary.

- Before you start the interview, know as much as you can about what happened. Keep an open mind. Recognition is dependent on willingness to entertain the possibility of sexual abuse.
- See the child alone before the offender is seen, if possible. This facilitates the interview with the offender.
- Avoid interviewing the child in front of the parents. This may cause the child to seal over or expose the child to undue stress if parental reactions are initially strong and anxiety-ridden, or if the child contradicts the adults' history. The exception is the very young toddler, where separation increases anxiety.
- Determine the child's understanding of the purpose of the interview. The child has probably been questioned by various other authorities who fulfill a different role. *Keep the number of people who interview the child as low as possible.*
- Provide a *brief* description of your role and the purpose of this evaluation. Be certain to keep the child's level of cognitive development in mind. Inquire as to whether the child has already been told something about the interview:

Example: "I am a social worker who works in this department" is not a meaningful explanation to a 4-year-old.

Example: "Did your mommy tell you why you were coming here today?"

- With the presenting symptoms in mind, proceed slowly with some open-ended questions related to the alleged sexual abuse.

Example: "I understand you were upset after your baby-sitter left the other night. Can you tell me more about that?"

Example: "Your mommy tells me she brought you to the doctor because your pee-pee was hurting you. What happened when she brought you there? Can you tell me how it was that your pee-pee got hurt?"

- Move from *open-ended questions* to a *more narrow, direct focus*. Move step by step, as if you are closing a wide-angle lens to a more specific area. Take your time. Rushing will not assist. Direct questions are not synonymous with leading questions. They are simply moving you to a very specific area of inquiry.

Example:
- Acknowledge that a "hurt" happened.
- Inquire about how it happened: who was with the child?
- What were the circumstances around this happening: time, place, duration, onset, exchange of words or explanations, threats, bruises, coercion, affective and cognitive experiences, and other circumstances?
- Assess the child's unique experience of the events.

- If necessary, use age-appropriate media: puppets, dolls (anatomically correct, if possible), picture drawing. Get to know the child's own terminology for body parts and sexual acts, and use these words to get information.
- Gather facts: where it happened, when, how long. Where were the other family members? How was secrecy requested and enforced?
- If you fail to bring up the material, the child may assume there is something wrong and fear exposing it or think that it is not taken seriously.
- Always avoid "why" questions (e.g., "Why didn't you tell someone?" "Why did you let him?").
- Ask about siblings (i.e., were they abused?) and any other experiences of sexual activity with other adults. Sexually

abused children are vulnerable to revictimizations. Asking about siblings or other incidences may avoid guilt for harboring this information.
- Inquire gently about how the child's compliance was gained. Secrecy is an integral component to the sexual abuse dynamics. The most consistent impression children harbor is one of danger and fearful outcome based on secrecy. Their fears may be generated in such statements as the following:

Example: "This is our little secret so don't tell anyone; no one else will understand."

Example: "If you try to tell anyone, no one will believe you."

Example: "Don't tell your mother, she will hate you, she will hate me, she will kill you, she will kill me, it will kill her, she will send you away, she will send me away, or it will break up the family and you'll end up in an orphanage" (12).

- Threats of loss of love or loss of the family are often more frightening to a child than threats of violence.
- Do not introduce the specific names of any suspected offenders. First, make a general inquiry.

Example: "Has someone been touching or playing or doing things with your pee-pee? Who is that? Anyone else? Can you tell me more about what he does or show me with the dolls?"

- If the child has not been able to offer the name of a specific offender, the alternative is to provide the child with a list of possibilities.

Example: "Has anyone been touching your pee-pee and causing it to hurt? For example, your friends at school or your mom or dad or one of your teachers? Or maybe someone else you know?"

This avoids a leading question—e.g., "Was it your daddy?"—and enables both you and the court to observe whether this child can discriminate between alternatives and specify from a range of possibilities. It is thereby less likely to be classified as "suggestive" or "leading the witness" to one specific response. Use the word "hurt" judiciously. Some children do not experience the activities as hurtful; similarly young children may equate "touch" with only fingers touching and not make the cognitive association to penis touching genitals.

- If you must ask a leading question, it is best to follow it with a nonleading question that provides the opportunity (from a legal perspective) for the child to clarify or refute what has just been posed.

Example: "Did your daddy ever hurt your pee-pee?"
"How did he do that?" (child indicates with dolls)
"I see, well, did your mommy or uncle or teacher or anyone else ever do that to you?"
"How about your friends or brother?"

- Never condemn the offender or show any distaste for his behavior. Most children have affectionate ties to the offenders, or will interpret your condemnation as directed primarily toward themselves.
- Do not give up prematurely. Sexually abused children are often told not to tell anyone, or have important dynamic concerns that may hamper easy disclosure. Move circuitously and with encouragement and leeway, if necessary. Try sidestepping their dilemma by articulating it for them and validating their position.

Example: "Some mommies and daddies tell their kids not to

tell anyone. Then the kids don't know what they should do. Is that what it is like for you?"

Example: "Gee, when kids talk about their pee-pee's hurting it's usually because something has happened to them. It's very important we know about what happened so we can be of help and make sure it doesn't happen again."

An ambivalent therapist will not assist an ambivalent child. Disclosure is contingent on one's willingness to entertain the possibility of sexual abuse. Make it clear that you believe that talking is going to be helpful.

- Always take time to close the interview. Allow the child to ask you questions. Inquire about how the child feels about the revelation. Inquire about other worries or fears. Allow the child to know what will happen next, as much as possible. Praise the child for the disclosures and clarify any distorted notions—e.g., "You will not go to jail even though he told you that. He was wrong. You didn't do anything wrong."
- Irresolutions: Remember that facts may not entirely support or disprove the allegations. Don't assume unproved cases are unfounded. Victims are often more needy of support and assistance in unproved cases.

Mothers

In the older incest literature, mothers are seen as "pivotal" and as colluding with the abuser (15). Today there is growing awareness that there is a wide range of mothers in such situations. Some know about the abuse but are just as intimidated as the child or respond with "better this than leaving us." Others truly have no idea, are appalled at the revelation, and react appropriately to protect and support their child (10). Some form of denial is an almost universal finding in incestuous families. The initial reaction of shock and disbelief makes many mothers seem to lack the capacity to empathize with and support their child. If the mother knew about the abuse, one can assume she had psychodymanic reasons to live with the pathologic family homeostasis that is now challenged by the revelation. If she did not know, the revelation puts her into a very painful position. In cases of incest, she has to choose between her child and her partner. It cannot be stressed enough how difficult this choice can be. Situations in which a new partner, who represents a new chance, is found to be an abuser are often even more difficult than long-standing marital relationships that may already have been marred by chronic problems (10).

The literature describes incest mothers as having received poor mothering themselves and thus being unable to mother their children, after abdicating that role to one child (usually the oldest daughter). In the New England Medical Center study, 34 percent of the mothers reported they had been physically abused and 41 percent sexually abused in their own childhood. These research findings speak to the complexity of and the power of the intergenerational trend. What is not known yet is what differentiates those mothers who enter relationships with men who have abused their children from those who choose partners who do not. No correlation was found between particular diagnosis and types of reaction to the revelation. No significant difference was found between incest and non-incest mothers (10).

With nonjudgmental therapeutic intervention, many mothers can assume the role of protector and act appropriately.

Key Points for Interviews with Mothers

- Assess mother's ability to protect over time. Initial denial and ambivalence is expectable. The news is shocking and mothers need time, support, and helpful information to begin to integrate the unpleasant news.
- Individual counseling and advocacy is essential.
- An "auxiliary ego" can assist in containing and clarifying anxiety-ridden responses and confused notions, and assist in decision making and planning.
- When revealing confirmed allegations to the mother, *al-*

ways see the mother alone. Unbridled initial responses may subject the child to undue distress or may precipitate a retraction.

Offenders

Most critical to the impact of the trauma is the offender. Research has focused mainly on those who are jailed, which, although useful, does not address the wide range of psychopathology seen in clinical practice. Groth has made the important differentiation between the fixated and the regressed offender (13). The *fixated offender* is a pedophile whose psychosexual development is arrested and whose preferred sexual partners are children. Although these men may be capable of sexual relations with adults, this usually occurs as a means of reaching their partner's children. Pedophiles often have serial relationships with women who have children of the particular age range they favor. As soon as any suspicion is cast on them, they leave the family, city, or state, and begin elsewhere. They are only rarely seen in clinical practice because their pedophilia is usually ego-syntonic. Diagnostically they are found in all categories of the *Diagnostic and Statistical Manual of Mental Disorders, Third Edition (DSM-III)* (14).

The psychosexual development of *regressed offenders* does permit them to enjoy adult sexual relations, and they often are invested and caring parents. In times of stress, however, they resort to the less demanding sexuality offered by a relationship with a child: They enjoy and need the comparative power and the idealization. The cuddling aspect of the interaction feeds their pregenital needs, which can only be gratified in a relationship that also enhances their sense of authority and strength. What may begin as father–child closeness in a time of crisis (e.g., as when mother is hospitalized, or has a second job because father is unemployed) soon leads to genital arousal. At this stage offenders seem incapable of stopping themselves, and start abusing the child. Because of their inability to react empathically to their victim as a child, they fail to respond to the distress they provoke and later state that they would have stopped if the child had said no. They thus feel little personal responsibility.

Many regressed offenders are only marginally adequate adults with weak ego structures; they appear needy and empty in a psychiatric interview. They may be seen as benign and respectable in their environment, but can also be tyrannical within the home. They are invested in their families and often comply with therapeutic recommendations. Nevertheless, the potential for re-abuse, given conducive circumstances, is always present. Fathers who abused their children may become grandfathers who abuse their grandchildren.

Other categories of offenders include those who are *psychopathic*, whose main goal is satisfaction of their incessant need for gratification. To them children are just one more object to satisfy pansexual needs, in the same category as male or female prostitutes, lovers, or spouses. These offenders, who may brutalize their whole family, are also often capable of presenting a trustworthy image to their environment. They may be very successful professionally, or they may have connections to the criminal world. They react to the allegation with outrage, bring forth character witnesses, appeal to political figures, and pass lie detector tests. They are a real challenge even to the seasoned expert, and may well succeed in intimidating those who want to help the child. Their posture, threats, or punishments at home can lead the victim to retract allegations, thus further complicating the task of those attempting to protect the child. Prognosis for rehabilitation is always guarded, as with all psychopaths.

The rare *psychotic* or *retarded offender* requires intervention to remediate the primary condition. The psychotic offender may be schizophrenic, manic, or depressed and may use the victim in ways particular to his delusional system (e.g., to "sacrifice" his daughter's virginity, or to expiate some guilt). Prognosis after treatment of the psychosis depends on character structure and family dynamics.

Offenders who are *alcoholics* often try to deny their responsibility by blaming their inebriated state. Addiction to immediate gratification of pregenital needs may well be a common factor, but does not resolve the issue of personal responsibility.

Juvenile offenders may have access to children as siblings, friends, or baby-sitters. Most of them are sexual abuse victims who have dealt with their history by identifying with the aggressor. Many adult pedophiles started abusing children as teenagers (13). Sibling incest takes many forms, from rape to a relationship meeting some of both children's needs for security and affection.

Key Points for Interviews with Incestuous Fathers

- See the father alone, and present knowledge of sexual contacts as relayed from the child.
- State your role and intentions of providing help.
- Remain unambivalent about your certainty that children do not lie about these matters.
- Clarify that this indicates a problem that can be helped.
- Assess nature of the contacts with the children, ability to control impulses, factors that inhibit or release such behavior, ability to cease behavior, willingness to pursue treatment, current psychological functioning.
- Circumvent any denial. Don't require any "admission of guilt or repentence," but offer services. Don't get pulled into debates about the verity of the incidents. Stand firm on offering help for this problem.
- Present information about next steps (e.g., father has to plan to leave for now or child needs to be protected).

FORMULATION AND DIAGNOSIS

Responding to a sexually abused child and the child's family requires work on several tracks, and does not follow the usual sequence of diagnostic evaluation–formulation–treatment planning–treatment implementation. Usually, the treatment begins with the first contact: The child and the family need crisis intervention. The diagnostic assessment goes hand in hand with a constant evaluation of the child's safety, which may require action before all the diagnostic work has been done.

As stated in the description of the family, offenders, nonoffending parents, and victims present with a wide range of symptoms. Diagnoses commonly found are posttraumatic stress disorder in the child and adjustment reactions in all family members. In addition, it is imperative to investigate areas of strength or pathology of a more chronic nature. This may not be appropriate or possible in the immediate crisis, which may lower ego functioning considerably, but is crucial for long-term planning. Siblings are important in the family dynamics and also need to be seen.

Crisis intervention is usually the first intervention needed (17, 18). After 6 to 8 weeks of crisis intervention, long-range plans may include individual or group therapy, or no therapy with periodic reassessment to allow the parents to consult with the clinician about their own anxieties and about the child's development.

Overall Goals

- Restore the family to a pre-crisis level of functioning, minus the incest.
- Prevent crystallization of psychological or psychosomatic symptoms into long-term adjustment problems.
- Detect patients predisposed to psychopathology and decompensation.
- Strengthen ability to cope with future stress by expansion of available repertoire of adaptive mechanisms.

Group therapy is particularly useful for members of incest families. Issues of social isolation, being "the only one," feeling out of step with peers, suffering from low self-esteem, depression, guilt, as well as practical life issues are more effectively dealt with in a group situation. Group therapy can be extremely useful for victims, mothers, siblings, *and* offenders (18).

Long-term consequences of sexual abuse are manifold, but not invariable. It is not clear why some abused children remain victims, whereas others perceive themselves as survivors (7). Intervention, including psychotherapy in childhood, will hopefully aid their development into survivors. Long-term outcome studies are yet to come.

RAPE

Rape of children, like sexual abuse, is a criminal act more frequent than once thought. For definitions and how they overlap, see the beginning of the chapter.

Presenting Complaint

Rape victims are often brought to an emergency room by their parents, who are as upset as or more upset than their child. The psychologic aspect of the trauma is often greater than the physical one. Although pedophiles may hurt their victims for gratification of sadistic impulses, most violence occurs as a means to gain the child's compliance, and is usually less severe than in adult rape.

Childhood rape is usually disclosed by the child. In younger children, conflict about disclosure is related to their relationship to the offender: If there is none, there is less conflict. In older children, particularly adolescents, revelation of rape may be impeded by the same issues as seen in adult victims: self-recrimination, guilt, fear of being blamed or seen as "dirty," and fear of retaliation from the rapist.

Parental reactions vary from anxious disbelief, to denial, to panic.

Clinical Intervention

Medical, psychiatric, and legal interventions need to be coordinated. A *medical examination* of the child is essential, and should be performed by a pediatrician comfortable with such exams, and willing to testify in court if necessary. As with adult victims, the gathering of corroborating data is an essential part of the medical exam: The medical record should be written as if ready for court.

A gynecological exam should be performed in the context of a general medical exam, and only after establishing a relationship with the child. Performing an internal exam on an uncooperative, panic-stricken child is a retraumatization that is never justifiable. If the exam cannot be delayed, it should be performed on a tranquilized or even anesthetized child. Hospitalization may be necessary.

A comprehensive physical exam includes the following:

- Medical history, including gynecological history if appropriate.
- History of the assault, recorded in a legible, precise, and nonprejudicial manner.
- Recording of all observations on how the victim presents.
- Physical examination, noting all signs of physical trauma, described in words as well as on a body chart.
- Collection of medical–legal evidence (e.g., semen, blood, any foreign matter, loose hairs).
- Pelvic examination and collection of lab specimens (e.g., for evidence of sexually transmitted disease).
- Medical therapy, if necessary, for physical injuries, pregnancy, or sexually transmitted disease.
- A rape kit, as used for adult victims, should be available.
- Follow-up is always necessary.

Psychiatric intervention should occur concurrently with the medical examination. Basic information and interviewing techniques are described in the paragraphs on sexually abused children.

Particular to rape victims is that they are being seen after an assault that has interrupted the flow of their usual life. The victim and the victim's family may have been functioning very well, adequately, or poorly before the rape. When seen in the emergency room they are in a state of crisis, and need to be responded to on that level: The parents' level of functioning may be seriously compromised and they need pragmatic guidance as well as support. There are no predetermined family patterns related to the rape of a child, but some children are more likely to be raped than others: those who have been sexually abused before, are lonely and needy, or have poorly developed social or cognitive skills and cannot respond with adequate suspicion and self-protectiveness. These children may become victims of strangers or of peers.

The victim and the family's tendency is to look for a cause, which easily leads to blaming the victim ("if only . . . "). A child may be overtly blamed or punished for the rape when the parents cannot tolerate their helplessness or rage toward the offender. This requires intervention: No misbehavior or breaking of rules makes the child responsible for being raped. Intervention decreases the potential for the revictimization of the child.

Another relatively common finding is a reaction of overprotectiveness toward the child, sometimes with paranoid tendencies, which can be quite regressive and allow latent pathology to surface (e.g., school phobia).

All parents have fears about the effects of the rape on the child and the whole family. Their anxiety has to be listened to without the child being present.

Legal Issues

The requirements vary from state to state. In Massachusetts, a report to child protective services has to be filed if the parents are not capable of responding adequately to their child, and should be filed if services can thus be secured for the family. Criminal reporting and prosecution is separate from child protective service intervention. If the offender is a person the child will continue to see (e.g., if the offender lives in the neighborhood or goes to the same school), involving the police may be necessary and helpful.

Treatment Planning

Pre-rape levels of functioning vary greatly, as do diagnoses. Some children exhibit a rape trauma syndrome similar to the one described in adults (19). Others may respond with behavior symptoms, or minimal symptoms. The level of parental anxiety strongly affects the child's reaction.

The first therapeutic intervention required is crisis intervention: Individual meetings with the victim and individual couple meetings with the parents are necessary. Whether long-term therapy is necessary has to be decided in the course of crisis intervention.

Conclusion

The recent dramatic increase in reported sexual abuse challenges psychiatry with new issues. On a practical level, the need to cooperate with other agencies and in particular with the legal system conflicts with the traditionally more passive and isolated role of the psychotherapist. On a theoretical level, many questions arise. Is sexual abuse always linked to later psychopathology? Why do some victims identify with the aggressor, whereas others internalize a victim identity? What is the importance of trauma in human development? What are the costs and benefits of intervention?

References

1. Bourne R, Newberger E: "Family autonomy" or "coercive intervention"? Ambiguity and conflict in a proposed juvenile justice standard in child protection. Boston University Law Review 57:670–706, 1977

2. Chapter 288 of the Acts of 1983, amending section 51B of Chapter 119 of the General Laws of Massachusetts

3. Sgroi S: Handbook of Clinical Intervention in Child Sexual Abuse. Lexington, Mass, DC Heath & Co, 1982

4. Katan A: Children who were raped. Psychoanal Study Child, vol 28, 1973

5. Gutheil T, Avery N: Multiple overt incest as family defense against loss. Family Process 16:1, 1977

6. Herman J, Hirschman L: Father Daughter Incest. Cambridge, Harvard University Press, 1981

7. Tsai M, Feldman-Summers S, Edgar M: Childhood molestation: variables related to differential impacts on psychosexual functioning in adult women. J Abnorm Psychol 8:4, 1979

8. Kinsey A, et al: Sexual Behavior in the Human Female. Philadelphia, WB Saunders Co, 1953

9. Finkelhor D: Sexually Victimized Children. New York, Free Press, 1979

10. Gomes-Schwartz B, Horowitz J, Sauzier M: Sexually Exploited Children: Service and Research Project. Washington, DC, U.S. Dept. of Justice, 1984

11. Massachusetts Department of Social Service Statistics, 1984

12. Summit R: The child sexual abuse accommodation syndrome. Child Abuse Negl 7:177–193, 1983

13. Groth N: The incest offender, in Men Who Rape. New York, Plenum Press, 1979

14. American Psychiatric Association: Diagnostic and Statistical Manual of Mental Disorders, Third Edition. Washington, DC, American Psychiatric Association, 1980

15. Kaufman I, Peck A, Tagiuri C: The family constellation and overt incestuous relations between father and daughter. Am J Orthopsychiatry 24:266–279, 1954

16. Bender L, Blau A: The reaction of children to sexual relations with adults. Am J Orthopsychiatry 22:500–518, 1937

17. Simrel K, Berg R, Thomas J: Crisis management of sexually abused children. Pediatr Ann 8:5, 1979

18. Burgess A: Sexual Assault of Children and Adolescents. Lexington, Mass, Lexington Books, 1978

19. Sauzier M: Emergency care of rape victims, in Emergency Psychiatry. Edited by Bassuk E, Birk A. New York, Plenum Press, 1984, pp 271–285

PART 3

CONSULTATION AND RELATED CLINICAL PROBLEMS

Chapter 12.	Consultations	243
Chapter 13.	Forensic Child Psychiatry	251
Chapter 14.	Adoption and Foster Care	269
Chapter 15.	Infant and Toddler Psychiatry	289
Chapter 16.	Genetic Issues in Child Psychiatry	303

Chapter 12

Consultations

Ourania Madias, M.D.

Kenneth S. Robson, M.D.

Consultation by child psychiatrists to a variety of professionals and institutions is a powerful and frequently used skill. In the broadest sense the consultant's role is *therapeutic*: Although not always involving direct clinical care, this process can often alter or improve the development-facilitating characteristics of settings and institutions serving children and their families. The child psychiatric consultant's role is also *political*: it can influence the policies and practices of courts, schools, social service agencies, and levels of funding as well as priorities for such funding in local, state, and federal legislatures (1–10).

Unlike its clinical counterpart, the consultant's role is complex in other ways as he or she encounters the issues involved in relating to larger systems, groups, and hierarchies, all of whom, while asking in some way for expert guidance, will resist or actively discourage receiving such guidance and the physician bringing it. It may be useful, as Jellinek (11) pointed out, to enter the consultative setting with the expectation of being unloved, an outsider bringing more work for the consultee, a threatening and overpaid presence, and an expert who often must minimize his or her expertise. Indeed, the consultant, as in psychotherapeutic work, must attend to his or her powerful reactions to the experience. These often include discouragement or resentment at not being valued and appreciated, reactions based on one's personal past and grandiose perceptions of one's influence.

Nevertheless, whatever the setting, the consultant must begin with an empathic appreciation of the consultee's position and perspective. Only then can the consultant's expertise in clinical issues, development, group process, and political–institutional resources be utilized.

The Process of Consultation

Although the specific nature of the consultative task will vary according to setting, as discussed later in this chapter, there are some common elements to the process that are essential and practically useful to understand:

- Speak the "language" of the consultee; for example, pediatricians pressed for time will not be able to use a lengthy and anxiety-provoking psychodynamic explanation of patient and staff behavior. Such is even more the case with legislators and their aides.
- Become acquainted with the particular history and background of the consultee's setting (e.g., program details, prior consultation, prior and current personnel).
- Establish initial contact with whomever requests the consultation but be certain to connect with the system's leadership as well if not the initial source of the request (e.g., school principal, chief of pediatric service, judge of the court).
- Establish as clearly as possible from the outset "who wants what from whom" and at what rate. It is important to read between the lines in this regard to avoid being used to resolve internal systems problems and destroy the potential usefulness of one's role.
- Recognize the limitations of the consultation as early as possible. The achievement of modest, concrete goals often

is more effective in establishing alliances and a positive consultative "niche" than the promise of more grandiose services.
- Retain sufficient distance to avoid splitting in the consultative alliance. A rapport with only part of a system (e.g., the head nurse but not the attending on a pediatric service) often trades short-term comfort for long-term failure in the consultative task.

The basic *goals* of all consultations also involve common features in many respects parallel to therapeutic ones. These include:

- Establishing empathic contact.
- Facilitating growth-promoting processes (e.g., changes in behavior and awareness of nurse, physicians, teacher, or judge).
- Utilizing and calling on the inherent skills and capacities of the consultee, ultimately to become *less* rather than more important to that person, setting, or institution.

SPECIFIC TYPES OF CONSULTATION

Pediatric Consultation–Liaison

Initial consultation requests in pediatric settings often arise around:

- A particular patient problem, such as impulsiveness, noncompliance with regimens, or self-destructive risk.
- Differential diagnostic questions around somatoform disorders.
- Staff distress or concern about parent behavior (e.g., as with dying leukemic children or abused children).
- Requests for therapeutic intervention (e.g., psychoactive agents).

If the request involves patients or their families, it is essential that prior informing of the child or family take place to minimize defensiveness and splitting. Otherwise the psychiatrist's presence may be experienced as threatening, puzzling, or unwelcome. Direct, concise, concrete, and prompt feedback, both verbal and written, is essential in such situations if one is to be helpful. Overall, the Italian dictum *festina lente* (make haste slowly) is in order. However, the directions suggested by the consultant must be realistic and implementable within each particular pediatric setting. Awareness of staff emotional responses, as with a dying child or a sexually abusing family, may be central to effective responses to the consultation request, but tactful and understated explanations of such issues is critical.

In the best of circumstances, a well-crafted consultation to an individual patient problem may lead to more frequent requests and, ultimately, a more permanent liaison relationship with a ward, service, or subspeciality. Such connections can develop new clinical services (e.g., a Tourette's Clinic shared by child psychiatry and neurology, or groups for nurses, enhanced child psychiatric teaching in the pediatric curriculum, and additional funding of child psychiatric staff salaries).

School Consultation

Because the school is the work place of the child, and because increasingly available psychological services are being offered there (through PL94-142 [the law that mandates special services for children aged 3 to 21 with mental, emotional, or physical handicaps who require supplementary educational assistance] or local special educational and "mainstreaming" programs), the child psychiatrist must assume that contact with schools and school systems is an essential aspect of his or her role. Besides the formal contractual arrangements between a consultant and school system, common in clinical practice, establishing contact with the teacher(s) and school of one's own patients is often necessary and always useful; such episodic contact can develop into an influential intervention.

It is especially important to understand the basis of the

consultative arrangement within the school setting. If, for example, one is requested to evaluate individual children, are such evaluations to include family contacts? What safeguards exist to maintain confidentiality? To whom are you responsible? Is classroom observation acceptable to all faculty? How will you interface with existing staff psychologists or guidance counselors? Can you gain ready access to key members of the power structure (e.g., principal, superintendent)?

In asking and answering these questions, the consultant must keep in mind system, town, and district politics; funding issues and constraints; and the constant awareness that one is in an educational rather than a medical service delivery system. Flexibility and patience can lead to increasing energies at the administrative levels of the school system where more constructive change can be implemented.

Forensic Consultation

Child psychiatrists, in their clinical patient care as well as broader roles, are increasingly involved with courts, lawyers, and judges. Such involvement is sufficiently complex to require a chapter in its own right (see Chapter 13).

Adoption and Foster Care

The number of children involved in foster care and adoption is expanding. Many of these children are among the most seriously disturbed (see Chapter 14). Child psychiatrists can play a useful role in relation to adoption and foster care by consultation to agencies and institutions that serve such children and their families.

Agency Consultation

Within the current scene, the agencies empowered to care for children and their families are increasingly numerous and complex. These include state and local welfare systems, child care services (e.g., day care, group homes), residential settings, protective services, and advocacy structures. Several common problems appear to be present in these systems, as discussed below.

The roles of respective agencies are often redundant and the boundaries of mandate's blurred. For example, welfare, protective services, and mental health departments may all be responsible for intervention with and funding of varieties of troubled children. Who is "in charge" is often less clear.

"Therapeutic" services are increasingly present within agencies where this was not previously true (e.g., group homes, emergency shelters). Although such changes are primarily fiscal in origin, they complicate the life of the child psychiatrist consultant. The consultant may have *less* to say about major decisions affecting children's lives. For example, a child's length of stay in a group home or residential treatment center is no longer the domain of the child psychiatrist as therapist or case administrator. Many settings view their mandate as primary in a child's life; struggles between treatment programs, residences, and state agencies for control can lead to extremely complicated situations. In the area of custody and foster care, the consultant can see such dilemmas in operation.

Finally, the larger question of to what degree the agencies involved see themselves *in loco parentis* has begun to affect the consultative process and its problems. Agency interventions can frequently cause more difficulty than the initial clinical problem. (This situation can arise in incidents of alleged sexual abuse that immediately lead to family disruption, multiple losses, and related trauma.) The consultant needs to be aware of these issues in making effective interventions, acknowledging limitations within the consultative request, and advising or lobbying vis-à-vis political forces that shape agency policies.

Political Consultation

From the previous sections within this chapter it should be evident that the clinical arena is increasingly entwined in immediate and powerful political institutions and policies that *directly* affect questions of medical care and available services to children and families, reimbursement for these services, questions of professional competence and licensing, quality of care, viability of educational programs, and approval for necessary research studies.

Hence the child psychiatrist needs to appreciate the critical importance of his or her role as an advocate for children, families, and the professional agencies that serve them. Proactive involvement may be useful; passively ignoring such problems ensures further erosion of budgets and services essential for optimal levels of care for children who, of course, do not speak for themselves. The political consultant can perform a variety of tasks, including:

- Knowing and maintaining contact with key legislators (local, state, and federal) sympathetic to children's issues and needs.
- Testifying before legislative committees involved in decisions and policies affecting children.
- Writing letters to legislators and their staff vis-à-vis pending legislation.
- Educating legislators and their staff about the facts of many clinical situations; busy politicians make critical decisions on the basis of available knowledge (or supposition); *brief* fact sheets and personal contact can influence voting patterns and appropriations.
- Remaining available to run for office in professional societies or public sector settings where expert knowledge can influence policy directions and budgets.

REFERENCES

1. Ahsanuddin KM, Adams JE: Setting up a pediatric consultation-liaison service. Psychiatr Clin North Am 5:259–270, 1982

2. Berlin IN: Psychiatry and the school, in Comprehensive Textbook of Psychiatry III, Vol 3. Edited by Kaplan H, Freedman A, Sadock B. Baltimore, Williams & Wilkins Co, 1980, pp 2693–2706

3. Caplan G: The Theory and Practice of Mental Health Consultation. New York, Basic Books, 1970

4. Caplan G: Types of mental health consultation. Am J Orthopsychiatry 33:470–481, 1963

5. Koocher GP: Talking with children about death. Am J Orthopsychiatry 44:404–411, 1974

6. Lewis M: Residential treatment, in Comprehensive Textbook of Psychiatry III, Vol 3. Edited by Kaplan H, Freedman A, Sadock B. Baltimore, Williams & Wilkins Co, 1980, pp 2685–2692

7. Schowalter JE, Solnit AJ: Child psychiatry consultation in a general hospital emergency room. J Am Acad Child Psychiatry 5:534–551, 1966

8. Schowalter JE: Death and the pediatric house officer. J Pediat 76:706–710, 1970

9. Sherman M: Communicating: a practical guide for the liaison psychiatrist. Psychiatr Clin North Am 5:271–281, 1982

10. Bernstein NR, Sussex J (eds): Handbook of Psychiatric Consultation with Children and Youth. New York, SP Medical & Scientific Books, 1984

11. Jellinek M: Presentation to Child Psychiatry Board Review Course, Boston, Massachusetts, June 1985

Chapter 13

Forensic Child Psychiatry

Joseph J. Jankowski, M.D.

William P. Monahan, J.D.

Stephen Porter, M.D.

During the past 25 years there has been an increase in activity at the interface of child psychiatry and the judicial system. The dependent status of children (the term "dependent" in this instance is used as a legal term, not to be confused with the psychological definition of dependence or reliance) results in their vulnerability to both the emotional and legal problems that may occur within the family. It is often difficult to clarify children's legal rights from those of the parent and society. Only in this past quarter century have the unique emotional and developmental issues of childhood been seriously considered in assessing children's rights. This change has resulted in increased involvement of child psychiatric clinicians in the judicial system around issues of physical or sexual abuse, neglect, domestic violence, custody and placement, and the termination of parental rights.

In this chapter several problem areas relating to the legal rights of the child, the parent, and society will be reviewed and clarified. A format for the basic forensic evaluation will be presented, and special topics related to the evaluation will be examined in some detail.

Problem Areas in Forensic Child Psychiatry

Children's Rights

The areas that commonly involve children's rights are status offenses, commitment, psychotherapist–patient confidentiality, and informed consent.

Status offenses are acts committed by children or adolescents which would not be considered criminal if committed by adults. Children are assigned the status of minors, and under this status are considered to have obligations to their parents (e.g., to attend school, to be obedient). They are considered status offenders when they disregard the obligations of "minor status" and commit acts of truancy, ungovernability, and running away. Status offenders are children whose acts demonstrate social or emotional problems; often they are inappropriately criminalized.

Commitment of a child to a psychiatric hospital by a parent can take place with the help of a psychiatrist. In cases where commitment is indicated and parents refuse, a court hearing is requested to determine the existence of evidence to support nonadmission.

Therapist–child patient privilege is to be carefully protected. Generally, it can only be broken under two circumstances: if the child approves and in the event of a potential or actual threat to the loss of life.

Informed consent is complicated by the degree of adult status conferred on a child and the presumed and actual capacity for understanding with which the child is endowed. Recent judicial decisions have made changes in the following areas of informed consent:

Emergency Care. Twenty-nine states have statutes that explicitly permit medical treatment to be rendered to a minor without parental consent in an emergency, but *only* if the parent or guardian's consent cannot be obtained.

Substance Abuse. In Massachusetts a 12-year-old can receive medical treatment without parental consent for drug abuse if *two* physicians find that the minor is dependent on drugs. Most other states have no minimal age requirement. There is no provision for treatment of alcoholism without parental permission in most states.

Pregnancy Detection and Care. In 1979 the Supreme Court decided that minors who are mature and well informed can make a decision regarding abortion on their own. When children are not mature or of majority age (e.g., 18 or older, depending on state law) and cannot decide for themselves, a judge will decide for them on the basis of the child's best interest, not necessarily in consultation with the parents. In effect, the Supreme Court decided that when a family disagreement has occurred or is likely to occur, the state will assume the role of "parent" and decide when a child can be trusted to make an independent informed decision.

Voluntary Commitment. A parent or guardian's request for voluntary admission to (and discharge from) a psychiatric hospital is sufficient if the child is under 16 years of age. If 16, the child's request is sufficient. Before admission, the person making application (minor or parent) will be given the opportunity to consult with an attorney concerning the legal aspects of a voluntary admission.

Right to Refuse Treatment. The absolute right of any competent mental health patient to refuse medication, except in an emergency situation, has been established. The patient can be overruled only if determined to be incompetent, in which case it is required that, except in an emergency, a guardian must be appointed to make the decision on the patient's behalf.

It is worth mentioning a category of children for whom standard consent law matters. Children who are considered "emancipated" can give consent for medical, surgical, and psychiatric services in 37 states. Emancipated status is gained by reaching the age of majority, entering into a valid marriage, being on active duty in the military, or by judicial recognition of parent–child conduct that frees the child from the care, custody, and control of the parent. For example, the courts have ruled that if a child with parental permission moves out and lives on his or her own, the child is determined to be emancipated until and unless the parent consents, by judicial declaration; for example, in 18 states a minor can consent to diagnosis and consultation for mental and/or emotional disorders, and in all states a minor can consent to treatment of sexually transmitted disease as well as other diseases dangerous to the public health.

Delinquency

English common law held that children under 7 years of age could not commit a crime because they did not possess "mens rea," a guilty mind. Before age 14 they were presumed to be "doli incapax," incapable of entertaining criminal intent. As a result, English law required children over 14 to stand trial like adults and, if guilty, to serve penalties as criminals. Since the turn of the century, when the United States established the first juvenile court, the concept "parens patriae" (the courts would protect those without another protector) came to include not only abused, abandoned, and neglected children, but all children charged with violating laws who have not yet reached the age of majority. As a result, equity among the various needs of children was accepted, irrespective of the various activities that led to court involvement. Because the early juvenile court was viewed as a civil and not a criminal proceeding, the following procedural safeguards employed in criminal courts did not apply: right to jury trial, proof beyond a reasonable doubt, right to defense counsel, bail, avoidance of hearsay evidence, indictment by a grand jury, and open hearings. These procedural commissions were also justified on the basis of the juvenile court being rehabilitative rather than judging the child's guilt.

However, the Supreme Court stated in 1967 that "basic rights" must be applicable to juveniles under the Bill of Rights. These basic rights include: the right to counsel, to confront and cross-examine witnesses, to remain silent, to invoke a privilege against self-incrimination, to be presented with a timely notice of charges, to receive a transcript of proceedings, and to obtain appellate review.

Custody Placement

Until 1839, fathers held absolute rights to children predicated on the fact that they owned and managed all family property. Since 1839, the courts were granted the power to determine child custody for children under 7. By the 1960s, 90 percent of contested custody cases in the United States were decided in favor of the mother unless it was shown by overwhelming evidence that she was unfit. This changed following the "in the best interests of the child" rule, which allowed that mothers are the preferable custodians for children under the age of 4.

In 1964, the appointment of a Guardian Ad Litem (GAL) (1) in custody disputes began. Such guardians, appointed by the court to act in the best interests of the child, were expected to conduct a thorough evaluation of the custody issues and report their findings and recommendations to the court. They found that many mothers were being awarded custody even though they were not the more effective parent.

With an increased awareness by the GALs and courts that the child's needs should be paramount, the mother's domination over custodial decisions began to change in 1971 (1). At that time, a Missouri court in *Garrett v. Garrett* (2) awarded custody to a father in the absence of unfitness of the mother, stating that "the rule of giving the mother the preferential right to custody is predicated upon the acts of motherhood, not the fact of motherhood." The court went on to comment that "the tender years presumption should be discarded because it is based on outdated social stereotypes rather than rational and up to date consideration of the welfare of the children involved." Currently, the rights of parents are considered equal; neither parent is automatically assumed to be the preferred custodian, and "the best interest of the child" rule is utilized in resolving custody disputes.

Custody placement decisions are most often in legal proceedings involving delinquency, parental separation or divorce, neglect/abuse or abandonment, and the inability of a parent to care for the child because of severe mental illness, physical illness, or death. Table 1 specifies the courts–agency involvement, the parent's rights, and the child's rights in the areas of child custody placement.

In 1974, the American Bar Association approved the Uniform Marriage and Divorce Act (3), which contained three proposals to improve the current practice of custody proceedings. They included:

- Access to litigation to modify custody is prohibited for 2 years after the issuance of a custody decree of evidence of serious harm to the child.
- The court may appoint for the child his or her own attorney who has more prerogatives than the GAL.
- The court may order a custody investigation, including professional consultation.

Custody placement decisions are most often needed in legal proceedings involving delinquency, parental separation or divorce, neglect/abuse or abandonment, and the inability of a parent to care for the child because of severe mental illness.

Termination of Parental Rights

Unlike custody and placement evaluations where the psychiatrist can function as a mediator to protect and preserve a child's access to both parents, in termination of parental rights cases the psychiatrist is expected to consider a permanent separation that might result in pain and suffering for both parents and children. The child psychiatrist's actions should take into account this potential outcome as well as the knowledge that the *greatest* suffering occurs when children are left in the uncertain limbo of prolonged foster care and deprived of the opportunity to have a permanent and stable home.

Evaluation for the termination of parental rights begins because of serious allegations of abuse and neglect. The involve-

Table 1. Child Custody Placement Decision Making

Decision	Court–Agency Involvement	Child's Rights	Parent's Rights
Delinquency	Places child in custody of state or back with parents, depending on severity or recidivism of act.	Treatment program where rehabilitation is planned. Assignment of a probation officer who oversees rehabilitation and makes all efforts to return and maintain child with parents.	Few rights in juvenile court until hearing. After hearing, right of appeal of decision. Visitation privileges at facility or home.
Separation or Divorce	Orders forensic evaluation in contested custody case. Assignment of custody dependent on: • continuity of case, age, sex, and development of child • capacity at present to be aware of child's needs • ability to allow the other parent to co-parent • ability to provide for child physically and emotionally and medically	Visitation with noncustodial parent unless circumstances indicate otherwise.	Contest custody of child. Equal rights of custody.
Long-Term Temporary Placements	Do not serve child's best interest		

ment of multiple social agencies, placement in foster care, and prior testimony in court has often taken place. There has been an attempt at a therapeutic intervention at the individual or family level (involving visitation between child and parent and psychiatric treatment of the parent and/or the child) prior to involvement of the child psychiatrist as evaluator at the termination of parental rights.

The evaluation process requires a careful orchestration of the involved parties so that they can consider what is in the best interests of the children. It is especially important for the child psychiatrist to clarify his or her mandate, to act and to make certain of access to the information and persons necessary to make an assessment of parental fitness.

Given the seriousness with which our courts view government interferences into the privacy of family life and the irreversible changes that may result, the laws and evidenciary issues involved in terminating parental rights are far more strict than in some cases involving disputed custody and placement. Custody placement decisions are rendered by a judge based on "preponderance of the evidence." This standard of proof requires a simple majority of the evidence. In sharp contrast, the Supreme Court in 1982 (4) established that a parent's right may only be terminated if parental failure can be proven "by clear and convincing evidence." In addition, it has been required that proof of parental unfitness be current and continuing at the time of the hearing. It is imperative that the child psychiatrist carefully conduct the evaluation to determine the level of parental fitness.

THE FORENSIC EVALUATION

The child psychiatry forensic evaluation is a psychiatric evaluation of parents and children conducted expressly for the court (5–10).

Forensic child psychiatric evaluations differ from traditional clinical evaluations in the following ways:

- Patients (any member of the immediate family) do not usu-

ally initiate forensic evaluations, but instead perceive participation as part of impending legal proceedings.
- Patients are not seeking care for a symptomatic interpersonal or intrapsychic problem, but because of an unresolvable conflict with a family member or a human service agency.
- Evaluators must collect more extensive data to ensure objectivity of historical, subjective, and ancillary data.
- Investigation usually takes 3 to 6 months or more and includes comprehensive testing.
- Interviews are conducted with child, parents, and all relevant ancillary sources.
- Home visits are routinely included.
- Mediation and arbitration of adversarial relationships between parents, agencies, and the courts must be dealt with before proceeding with the evaluation.
- Psychological, educational, and medical assessments of all relevant family members with "expert clinician" input for special problems are routinely included when indicated.

The first step of a forensic evaluation is to clarify the issues to be addressed and to map out a strategy that will allow for an effective evaluation. Factors to consider include:

- origin of the requested consultation
- appropriateness of the case
- for whom will the evaluator work
- to what ends will the evaluation and resulting reports be used.

A common misconception is the unrealistic expectation as to the rapidity with which the forensic evaluation should determine parental fitness or develop complicated custody and visitation arrangements. A few meetings with the concerned parties are insufficient. In addition, the psychiatrist cannot evaluate individuals who refuse or are resistant to participate.

Some important considerations before beginning a forensic evaluation are as follows:

- A forensic evaluation cannot be used as an emergency intervention.
- Forensic evaluations require a lengthy process because of the seriousness of the issues and potential long-term consequences of the recommendations.
- Cases that involve a conflict of interest, such as a potential or business relationship with one of the involved parties, should not be accepted.
- Cases that provoke intense countertransference reactions that may result in biases should be refused.
- Once an agreement on your role as forensic evaluator is reached, it is important to write out the terms and fees for this service and distribute them to all parties for confirmation and ongoing references.
- A careful, thoughtful, and comprehensive report is a necessary product of any forensic evaluation.
- If testimony in court is required, it should be established at the convenience of the evaluator.

Forensic Evaluation Guidelines

- Maintain a child-centered focus. The child psychiatrist's role is to determine what is in the best interest of the child who is being considered.
- Assume a nonadversarial role. This enables the child psychiatrist to be effective during all phases of a forensic intervention: arbitration, mediation, and reconciliation.
- Attain designation as an evaluator for the court even though a specific party may make the referral or pay for the evaluation.
- Avoid the inclination to become the therapist. Detailed interviews are needed to obtain information for decision making, but they should remain in the realm of data collection, not treatment.
- Delineate the role of each member of the clinical evaluation team (if a team approach is utilized) before the team evaluation begins. Evaluations can be performed by one clinician or by a team, depending on clinical circumstances and staff availability.

- Include recommendations for child and parents based on clinical information.

Given orders by the court, patient compliance is rarely a problem. If it is, the uncooperative patient's attorney or court can be notified in writing and asked to intervene. If lack of compliance continues after this notification, the evaluation is sent to the court in an incomplete form, including all findings available up to that point but without a decision. A decision cannot be rendered until all information is complete. The court can either order the patient to complete the evaluation or utilize their noncompliance as a factor in its decision.

Special Issues

Consultation

Consultation allows the forensic child psychiatrist to be of assistance to courts, attorneys, parents, children, and human service agencies by clarifying chemical and legal issues. Guidelines for consultation are given below.

- If complete information is not available at the point of referral, a comprehensive forensic evaluation should be recommended before a specific course of action is suggested.
- If there is insufficient evidence to pursue court proceedings, the consultee should be advised to hold off further action or to pursue a different course.
- It is recommended that the psychiatrist request appointment as a neutral evaluator by the court with the agreement of all parties.
- All consultation efforts should be formalized with written reports sent to the consultee. These will become part of the historical content of this case, whatever the outcome.
- Forensic child psychiatry consultants often serve as brokers between parents, attorneys, courts, and psychiatric clinicians. They help clarify how cases might be approached clinically and legally.

- Reports written for the court are the tangible end product of a forensic evaluation and serve as the basis of all related testimony.
- The report should be written in a clear, concise, organized narrative style that places events in a coherent sequence.
- The personality or behavior of an individual should not be described with jargon, diagnostic labels, or interpretive comments.
- When appropriate, the child's specific reactions should be described and compared with those that might be expected of a normal child at a similar developmental stage.
- The report's description of events, problems, and behavior should be logically organized so as to support its conclusions. Specific sections may be used to highlight specific aspects.

Report Writing

Remember that the report is written for nonmedical persons who wish to use a psychiatric opinion to help solve a legal problem. The following items should be included:

- Identifying data—including names and birth dates of all patients and the specific court involved.
- Introduction—including a statement of the problem, source of referral, specific contacts with all parties, and a description of all materials reviewed in preparation of the report.
- History and problems as viewed by mother.
- History and problems as viewed by father.
- Interviews with parents.
- Interviews with child or children.
- Home visits to both parents.
- Interviews with collateral sources—including interviews with teacher, guidance counselor, grandparents, other relatives, foster parent, agency staff, therapists, and physicians.
- Reports (includes reports from school, physicians, psychologists, and others).
- Findings specific for each person (e.g., each parent and child).

- Recommendations specific for each person.
- Rationale for recommendations (i.e., summary of case with rationale for decision).

Once the report is completed, draft copies are sent to each party before it becomes final. Once the parties have the opportunity to correct factual material and to clarify statements and relevant findings, the report is sent to the court.

Testimony

Mental health professionals often fear the court experience and frequently ask, "What should I say, or not say, and what will they ask me?" Their fear is exaggerated by the lack of supervised court experiences during their training. Frequently, the clinician's first experience in court occurs when his or her own therapy patient is involved in a court preceeding and the clinician is called to give an expert opinion about the patient's clinical functioning.

Expert opinion is generally sought on subject matter not within the ordinary experience of the court. In order to testify as an expert, there must be preliminary inquiry by the court concerning the expert's skill and knowledge of the particular subject matter. This is usually established by the testimony of the clinician with the aid of an attorney. The factual determination of whether or not the expert is properly qualified lies within the discretion of the trial judge.

The attorney who is presenting the expert is advised to focus on relevant professional education, training, and experience in his or her specialty area. The proposed expert's professional memberships, academic appointments, and relevant honors and awards can also be mentioned.

One cannot overemphasize the importance of good communication and prior discussion between the attorney and the expert witness before a court appearance. In some instances, the expert witness may be giving testimony about his or her own case and in others may be testifying as an expert in a case where the witness does not know the details about the patients involved but is asked to provide expert testimony about a specific subject (e.g., sexual abuse).

A suggested format for court presentation of a custody and visitation report is given below:

- Clinician should appear competent and self-confident when testifying in court.
- Language should be easily understood by everyone present and speech should be slow and clear.
- Remarks should be addressed to the judge, jury, and attorney asking the question.
- Opinions should be presented clearly and concisely.
- Qualifying and ambivalent statements should be avoided.
- Testimony should be organized in a narrative sequential style.
- Clinician may request that the attorney clarify a question not understood, request a brief recess to discuss the matter with a supporting attorney, or review his or her notes or report if unclear on an issue.
- A clinician who does not know the answer to a question or does not have an opinion on a specific matter may state so if this is the case.
- Expert witness should be familiar with and aware of all the issues involved in the testimony.
- Expert witness should review all dispositions (a series of questions directed to any or all parties by the attorneys prior to court) and be familiar with his or her own written report.
- When testifying on direct examination (questioned by the supporting attorney who has asked the clinician to testify), answer the questions as asked (do not become loquacious), and always try to end your testimony on a positive note.
- When being cross-examined (questioned by the attorney on the other side), be polite, cooperative, and straightforward, and do not create an oppositioned manner.

Monitoring

The recommendations for a case monitor to be appointed after the court decision can be crucial in determining the future course of the case. It is often the only way an evaluator can be certain that his or her recommended plan will be followed. Monitoring provides the capability to maintain continuity and modify decisions that might become outmoded with time and changes in circumstance.

The original forensic evaluator, who has the most information, is best suited for the role of the monitor. However, in some instances, it is not appropriate for the evaluator to continue as monitor if one of the parties considers the evaluator to be biased. It is important that the monitor be appointed by the court and acceptable to all parties.

The monitor's role is to serve the best interests of the child. This primary focus must be maintained despite the fact that the monitor may spend time guiding and supporting parents. Loss of focus can be avoided during the monitoring phase through regular visits with the child.

As the child grows and develops, needs change, requiring alterations in the relationship between the child and the parents. The monitor must mediate, educate, and counsel the parents to help them support their child's growth. The monitor might be called on to make decisions involving changes in visitation, physical custody, or placement itself.

The monitoring process is similar to psychotherapy except for the utilization of more direct recommendations and confrontation of the parent.

Monitoring may continue for a short (1 year or less) or lengthy (15 years or more) period of time, depending on the clinical needs of the case. In most instances, the children are stabilized after a year but the parents continue to require monitoring because of their own long-term conflicts. If unresolved conflicts that negatively affect the child continue or develop between the parents during the monitoring phase, it is recommended that the monitor send a formal report to the court explaining the problem and recommending a course of action.

A child psychiatric clinician is best suited by training and tradition to provide the monitoring process in forensic cases. An important distinction exists between attorneys and clinicians. Attorneys settle disputes and provide follow-up if called on regarding additional issues or new disputes. On the other hand, a clinician naturally provides follow-up as an integral aspect of clinical work.

Summary

The child psychiatrist must remain unbiased and open to all data available. Preconceived notions or decisions based on inadequate or premature data are not acceptable.

The time frame for any evaluation must be open-ended and reflect the needs of the case clinically being determined by the evaluator. Courts are generally understanding; attorneys and patients often are not. Also, a patient may wish to speed up or postpone the evaluation for his or her own benefit.

The child's best interest are to be served. Decisions regarding custody and placement are temporal; that is, they can be changed at any time, depending on clinical circumstances. This must be kept in mind as one struggles to serve the child's best interest at a particular time. Decisions are therefore cross-sectional; they reflect the here and now but may not predict what will happen in the future. The clinician evaluator's approach must be flexible, with the realization that the outcome or needs of the case may be different after several years.

Parents change with time and circumstances. Such changes need to be considered during the monitoring phase and incorporated in alterations of the initial decisions and court order. We do not live in a static world; there is no reason to believe that our decisions should be static. We can only make the best decision possible, given all available data at the time of the evaluation.

References

1. Hansen RW: Guardian ad litem in divorce and custody cases: protection of the child's interests. Journal of Family Law 4:182–184, 1964

2. Garrett v. Garrett, 464 SW 2d 740 Miss 1971

3. Foster HH Jr: Divorce reform and the uniform act. Family Law Quarterly 7:179–210, 1973

4. Santosky v. Kramer, 455 US 745, 769–770, 1982

5. Schetsky DH, Benedek EP (eds): Child Psychiatry and the Law. New York, Brunner/Mazel, 1980

6. Slovenko R: Law and Psychiatry. Boston, Little, Brown and Co, 1974

7. Stone A: Mental Health and the Law: A System in Transition. New York, Jason Aronson, 1976

8. Gutheil TG, Appelbaum P: Clinical Handbook of Psychiatry and the Law. New York, McGraw-Hill, 1983

9. Sandoff RL: Forensic Psychiatry: A Practical Guide for Psychiatrists and Lawyers. Springfield, Ill, Charles C Thomas, 1975

10. Goldstein J, Freud A, Solnit AJ: Beyond the Best Interests of the Child. New York, Free Press, 1973

Chapter 14

Adoption and Foster Care

Steven L. Nickman, M.D.

Marie Armentano, M.D.

Adoption

Approximately 1.5 percent of children in the United States are adopted by parents to whom they are unrelated by blood; another 1.5 percent are adopted by a stepparent or blood relatives. Studies (1, 2) suggest that the child psychiatrist will encounter adopted children (primarily those unrelated to their adopters) out of proportion to their prevalence in the population.

Until the early 1970s, most children placed for adoption were white infants. Societal changes have profoundly affected the pattern of adoption in America. Increased availability of contraception and abortion and lessened stigma for unmarried mothers who keep their babies have caused a "baby famine," and led to the emergence of hitherto unfamiliar forms of adoption. The definition of an "adoptable child" has undergone a radical broadening in response to pressure from would-be adopters, and with the support of social work professionals who have pioneered new kinds of placement (3). These include:

- Transracial adoptions
- Transnational adoptions
- "Special-needs" or developmentally disabled children
- Adoption of older children
- "Legal risk adoption"
- "Open Adoption"
- Increased adoption of black children by black families

Other changes include state subsidy of placement in recognition of certain children's unusual needs, and a greater acceptance of "nonmainstream" adoptive parents. Single persons, couples past childbearing age, and gay individuals are increasingly regarded as potential adopters.

Most adoptive parents cannot procreate. They have suffered a complex loss involving body image and identity as members of a genealogic chain (4). Nonmainstream adopters may have sustained similar or other losses. Society exerts pressure on couples to have children and encourages adoption when procreation is impossible, yet there is a subtle undercurrent of prejudice against adoptive families and adopted children (5). The adoptive process is affected by these stresses (4–6).

Factors Affecting Personality Development in Adoptees

Prenatal care and inherited constitution. Most important is the possibility of poor nutrition or substance abuse during pregnancy, affecting biologic substrates for cognition. (Heritability of intelligence and of psychiatric disorder are accepted to some extent by placement workers, but rarely preclude adoption because many workers and parents believe strongly in environmental influences.)

Early infant–caretaker interactions. Some children have had "good enough" experiences in infancy, with biological mothers or during brief fostering and after placement in adoptive homes. The greater the number of disruptions a child undergoes, the more likely it is that later personality formation will be affected. The later the adoptive placement, the more difficult the "take." Acting out in child and adolescent adoptees may be related to Winnicott's theory relating the "antisocial tendency" to early discontinuities in experience.

Adopter–adoptee relationships. Procreators "have" a child; adopters "get" one. The "gotten" child may be experienced as alien. Parents may have little support to cope with such feelings (6). Likewise, when an infant or toddler shows a grieving reaction for what is lost, this may be misinterpreted as rejection of the new parent. Adoptive ties may need help to get off to a good start.

"Telling," status losses, and fantasy formation. This factor is described later.

Adolescence and entry into adult life. Many young adoptees speculate about birth-parents and whether to seek them out. They may experience themselves as incomplete without such knowledge. In response to pressure from adoptees, many birth-parents, and some adoptive parents, bills have been introduced into state legislatures to make original birth certificates available to adoptees at age 18. Four states now have such laws; five have partial "mutual consent" laws. Opposition to reform is vigorous, and appears to come largely from adoptive parents. Adoption professionals are divided, but increasingly recognize the legitimacy of pressures for change (3, 7).

Clinical Interventions with Adopted Children

Child psychiatrists may be approached at various stages of an adoptive placement. Requests include:

- intervention around the adoptive process,
- assessments shortly after a child is placed in a home, and
- requests for advice or psychotherapeutic help in established adoptive families.

The first type of request has resemblances to the divorce-custody evaluations with which child psychiatrists are familiar; the last is similar to traditional office or clinic practice.

Intervention Around the Adoptive Process

This may involve a request by a court, social service agency, prospective adoptive parents, or an attorney to assess a child, a birth-mother, or the quality of the bond between a child and foster parents who hope to adopt. The child psychiatrist brings expertise to bear on emotionally charged areas in which hard scientific evidence is still scant. A written report or court testimony may be requested.

The child psychiatrist need not assume more responsibility than his or her experience warrants. If the child psychiatrist has substantial knowledge of child placement, placement-related recommendations can be incorporated into the report with greater confidence than would be the case with a less experienced psychiatrist. The latter, however, can still help by reporting clinical observations and providing diagnostic assessments. Ultimately the responsibility for placements belongs to the placing agency and the court.

Requests may be for assessments of individual children or sibling groups, or (more commonly) they may involve evaluation of child–adult interactions or of parental capability in the context of a "bonding study" or a court case involving the rights of a biological parent (8, 9).

Clinical assessment of children. Questions raised include the suitability of a child for adoption, as opposed to long-term foster care or group placement; less frequently, the appropriateness of placement in a specific family is considered. These questions are not usually posed "up front." Agencies do not assume that psychiatrists are expert in placement issues and those questions may emerge in discussion when a child is referred for evaluation. The clinician needs to know the child's full background. When practical, the prospective adoptive parents should be met and the clinician should request access to the agency's home study because assessment of a child may be more useful in conjunction with knowledge of potential caretakers.

The question for a psychiatrist, when considering "adoptability," is whether the child has sufficient emotional health to make use of a family as opposed to life in a foster or group home, which makes fewer demands for object-relatedness. This question is usually asked about children from 4 years old through adolescence, who have had substantial life experience and possibly neglect or abuse. Increasingly such borderline cases are tried in adoptive homes when the alternative is that the child will grow up essentially "objectless" in a series of foster placements or a group home.

Clinical procedure includes:

- Careful reading of the record, assessing developmental influences on the child.
- Full clinical evaluation, with special reference to the child's depth and style of relating.
- Referral for pediatric, psychological, and/or neurological evaluations when warranted.
- Observation of interactions between the child and the present caretakers.
- Full documentation of the clinician's observations, conclusions, and recommendations.
- Verbal contact with the referring placement worker, preferably in person.

Bonding studies and "rights of natural parent" situations. A situation that arises with increasing frequency is the so-called legal risk adoption in which a child who is not yet legally free for adoption is placed with a family that hopes to adopt that child, expecting that the court will abrogate the natural parents' right to the child based on past events. A child psychiatrist may be asked to assess the emotional bond between the child and the prospective adopters, and to establish whether it would be harmful to the child to be removed from present surroundings. This need arises when the birth-parent has shown a degree of interest that makes it impossible for the judge to terminate parental rights without hearing the case on its merits.

Another request may be to assess a birth-parent with respect to ability to be a caretaking or visiting parent to the child.

These situations constitute a new and complex challenge to law, custom, and the mental health professions. "Permanency planning," as now promoted by child welfare agencies, encourages early placement of children in adoptive homes or early return to natural parents. Such treatment plans respond to important clinical findings (8, 9), but they also aid the public treasury because children in foster care are supported by public funds whereas adoptions are not usually subsidized.

The important difference between this type of court contest and divorce custody litigation is that in the latter case the best interest of the child is virtually the only legal standard now in use; in contrast, although best interest is followed increasingly, many judges still use fitness of the natural parent as the more important standard (10). Biological ties may be deemed so important that unless a parent is unfit, the child's present attachments are given little weight. In the presence of different standards, one clinician is often not asked to evaluate all parties (as is the custom with divorce custody evaluations) because best interest may be addressed when dealing with the child and present caretakers, and fitness addressed when reporting to the court about birth-parents. Different experts may be asked to fill the two roles; clinicians who insist on retaining "impartial expert" status may be excluded.

Countertransference may interfere if the clinician has personal experience with adopting or with losing a child or has other personal feelings about such situations, or if there has been a de facto abandonment of the child by the natural parent, which seems partly an agency failure. The clinician's heart may go out to the natural parent as victim, and the clinician may be less inclined to appreciate deficiencies. He or she may, instead, identify with the child's attachment to the prospective adopters.

With older children who retain emotional ties to parents who cannot care for them, the controversial alternative of "open adoption" is used in some situations. Many would formerly have been kept in long-term foster care. Open adoption implies that the child will have contact with the original parent while living in a stable adoptive home.

Adoptive parents entering such arrangements must be able

to feel secure in their roles. Some, because of their personal notion of parenthood, cannot raise a child under these conditions. Psychiatrists may be asked to make recommendations in such dilemmas. From the standpoint of the child's welfare, the psychiatrist may be the only advocate of continued relationship with an emotionally impaired parent. A significant arguing point in favor of open adoption is that complete loss of a prior caretaker may be unfair to the child and may even make it harder for the child to commit to a new home.

Paramount in the consideration of return to parental custody, or continued relationships with birth-parents, are the following questions:

- Has the child shown evidence of regression or distress around the time of visits with biological parents?
- What interactions have been noted by observers during supervised visits?
- Would continued contact with a birth-parent be unacceptable to a preadoptive family with whom the child has a psychological right to stay?

Clinical procedure includes all the steps mentioned in the previous section. Additional procedures include the assessment of interaction and the assessment of parental capability.

Assessing interaction. This can be applied to child-with-prospective-adoptive-parents, as well as to child-with-birth-parents. The goal is to observe and describe what the child *does* and *seems to be feeling* in the presence of one or more adults, and vice versa, keeping in mind what would be expected developmentally considering the child's age and any existing neurologic or intellectual impairment. The adult should be invited to talk first with the psychiatrist. An invitation is issued to make use of the playroom and materials with the child in whatever way seems most natural. Assurance should be given of the clinician's awareness that this is a stressful situation. (This is indeed a stress interview, but parents have to cope with stress.) At times interaction with biological or prospective adoptive siblings is important to observe as well.

Relevant observations include: How often does the child approach the adult? How does the adult respond? Is there physical contact? Initiated by whom? How often? For how long? Is the adult alert to a young child's rapprochement behaviors, such as seeking eye contact, "checking back" for emotional refueling, and so on? Do the adult's facial expressions betray pleasure in the child? Do nonverbal cues match the emotional implications of words? Is the adult passive, controlling, or involved in comfortable mutuality while interacting with the child? Is the child's response to the examiner, a stranger, substantially different from the way the child behaves with the caretaker, or is there evidence of indiscriminate attachment?

The clinician should remain passive during the interview, but may need to facilitate interaction. The degree to which this is necessary should be noted.

A useful maneuver when assessing attachment in babies and younger children is to ask the adult to leave the room unobtrusively while the child plays. One then watches the child's behavior, including facial expression, whether attempts are made to find the adult, and how soon and persistently such attempts are made. Equally important is the child's behavior after the parent or parent-substitute is found. Does the child grin, with a decrease in bodily tension? Does the child seem indifferent? Does the adult seem confident, overly worried, or uninvolved during this procedure?

Assessment of parental capability. These evaluations may or may not progress to an interaction assessment as described above. Initially one interviews the adult, usually a biological parent from whom the child has been removed because of neglect or abuse. The format should be semistructured; several interviews may be necessary. Questions to be addressed include:

- Mental status, with particular reference to present level of functioning, intellectual and emotional. (Referral for psychological testing may be indicated if cognitive functioning

is in question, but projective testing is not generally necessary in these situations.)
- Attitude toward the child during pregnancy, neonatal period, and subsequently; expectations and hopes for the child's future.
- Community supports, including family, friends, social contacts, and religious contacts.
- Reality testing, including understanding of how the present situation came about; degree of insight versus projection of fault onto others.
- Understanding and knowledge of children's needs and development; specific knowledge of the child: What is at issue is the parent's ability to empathize with the child (e.g., to understand that important bonds may have been formed with foster parents). How narcissistic or self-serving is the parent's attitude? Is the child seen primarily as a separate person, an extension of self, someone who can help the parent in time of trouble, or a piece of property the parent has a right to control? Was the child's removal experienced primarily as a narcissistic blow or as the loss of a loved child? The ability to respond to specific factual questions about the child (e.g., what the child wants to become in adult life, or what activities the child presently enjoys) is often telling.

Assessment of other members of the adult's household, particularly new spouses or live-in friends. If the parent is found potentially capable, the next stage is observation of parent–child interaction. If visits have been ongoing, arranging this should not pose a problem. But if the child is in a preadoptive home, and visits with the natural parent have been cut off or allowed to lapse, the psychiatrist, along with the court and social service agency, must struggle with the question of whether to reopen the relationship.

Reports should be free of jargon and include illustrations and descriptions to support one's conclusions. Judgmental language should be avoided. The clinician should clear from the start as to who has a right to get copies of the report.

Requests to Assess a Child Soon After Placement

Often the covert message is: "Our whole family is having trouble since this child came to live with us. We aren't sure we can stick it out, but would feel terrible guilt if we decided not to keep him. Please help us figure out how to make things better, or how to bow out gracefully." Often the overt request is to assess a child's disturbance, with a view to possible psychotherapy. "Listening with the third ear" comes in handy at such times.

These situations need to be recognized for what they are—stages in a child's life when he or she exists, even if no longer in a legal limbo, then still in an emotional one. (The adoption may already have been finalized.) Parents may have been encouraged to "tough it out" by agency personnel, family, or friends, or may feel compelled to follow through on an initial commitment despite misgivings. Such considerations are especially relevant in the 1980s because of the increase in "new wave" adoptions involving older and traumatized children.

Include the following procedure:

- Obtain consent to talk to the placing agency.
- Catalyze creative working together of agency and family so they can together address whether the placement should continue.
- Remain available to see the child for extended evaluation, being open to hear parents' and workers' concerns.
- When necessary, help parents disengage from an initial commitment.
- In the event of disruption, maintain availability to all parties; offer to see the child again, and provide therapy or management as a valuable bridge.
- Remain alert to countertransference difficulties.

Requests for Help by Established Adoptive Families

Parents and children may deny the relevance of adoption to presenting complaints because of personal discomfort with the topic and because of society's lack of recognition of adoption as a stressor. Yet a disproportionate number of adopted children and adolescents experience difficulty. It seems wise to assume, until one is convinced otherwise, that adoption is an important issue. One wonders during the assessment of parents and child: How deeply should the psychiatrist inquire about adoption as a source of chronically injured self-esteem, in the face of initial denial?

Much attention has been paid to the identity problems of the adopted child, but little to those of the adoptive parent. Both have sustained losses. The therapist's role involves primary, secondary, and tertiary intervention:

Primary Intervention

The first aspect of primary intervention is conveying current knowledge to parents and pediatric colleagues concerning vulnerabilities of adoptive families, "age of telling," curiosity about birth-parents, the wish to search, and related issues.

With respect to age of disclosure about adoption, matters are no longer as clear as they seemed 20 years ago. The question of disclosure does not even arise with many children who are placed during the oedipal years and later, and who retain memories of their families of origin.

In the past 40 years, children placed as young infants or toddlers have traditionally been told of their adoption prior to age 4. Questions have been raised about this procedure. Cases are cited in which this knowledge interfered with developing self-esteem. Clinicians and parents should consider delaying disclosure until between the ages of 5 and 8. It seems likely that the extensive fantasizing and self-preoccupation that will follow such a revelation will be least detrimental to development after the oedipal period is largely resolved, and before the child must face the social and academic demands of the upper levels of elementary school.

Bearing in mind that telling is a process rather than an isolated act, we recommend that parents not enter into it out of a sense of urgency. They might wait until the child is conversant with the facts of reproduction and with the structures of society outside the family. A child might deal better with adoptive disclosure if the child can understand, "They were very young, had little money, and didn't believe they could take good enough care of you." This might mean waiting until age 5 or later, if the type of adoption and the parent's emotional, familial, and social situation permit. It can also mean the parents might have to tell a literal falsehood if at age 3, for example, the questions is asked: "Mommy, did I come out of your belly?" The emotional meaning of this question (i.e., "Am I really your child?") is what the boy or girl of that age needs an answer to. Yet to some parents it will seem highly unnatural to withhold the literal truth, even at an early age, and such parents may need help in tailoring their early revelations to their child's capacity to hear.

Concerns about original parents need to be dealt with. Such questions are legitimate and deserve to be answered with factual material. But it must be recognized that they also often represent the adopted child or adolescent's way of expressing normal impulses to individuate or to rebel. The response, "I'll help you search," may be given in anger and may arise from the parent's own insecurities. In such circumstances it is equivalent to the hostile retort to a child who threatens to run away: "I'll help you pack your bags." But it may be experienced as profoundly reassuring if a parent can say, "When you're 18, if you still wish, I'll try to help you find out who and where they are."

Identifying adoption-related elements in developmental crises of childhood. Nodal points may occur at which parents and children can be helped to become more comfortable with their feelings about adoption. Mild disturbances can be influenced in the direction of spontaneous resolution, rather than becoming entrenched as long-standing problems of adjustment.

Early identification of attachment problems. This is a supremely important task. Alert pediatricians and child psychiatrists can do a great service in this regard. Even in early placed children, cycles of mutual misunderstanding and rejection that lead eventually to serious conflict can be set up. In extreme cases, children placed in early infancy may be extruded by the family during adolescence.

Parents adopting older children are usually more prepared for problems with parent–child "fit" and may deal with them better. But infants may sense a discontinuity in their caretaking even before the conventionally recognized age for object constancy, and may respond by sleep, eating, or mood disturbances. Parents may be vulnerable and feel rejected. The clinician can explain that the child is mourning what has been lost, and that the parents are the best ones to help the child through it. Ongoing psychiatric advice may be required.

Secondary Intervention

When an adopted child becomes symptomatic to the extent that regular therapy is needed, feelings about adoptive status are high on the list of possible etiologic factors (1, 2, 7, 11). Many adopted children, particularly those in midlatency, demonstrate vulnerable self-esteem in relation to their knowledge of not having been kept by their birth-parents, experiencing themselves as cast-off or worthless. They may be moody, underachieve in school, or become aggressive. Psychiatric intervention can take as its goal the sensitive fostering of a grieving process so that the child can be freed-up to go on with the tasks of development. Responses need to be timed to a child's intermittent ability to bear painful affect. What is being grieved, in the case of early adopted children, is the fact that the child was not born into a family that wanted and could care for the child (11). With later-adopted children, object loss and various confusional states related to changes of caretaker also are involved. Some children feel stigmatized among peers because of adopted status, particularly if they appear foreign.

Parents who deal poorly with unpleasant feelings will need help in tolerating the sadness their child may express. "Isn't our love enough? Why does he have to keep thinking about those people he doesn't even know?" They might be encouraged to reflect on misfortunes they have experienced—particularly infertility, if present—to help them empathize with their child's pain (5).

The child can be encouraged to share fantasies of the original parents. Many adoptees fantasize extensively, and at times these fantasies crystallize into negative or shifting figures that maintain a hold on the growing child's imagination and influence in the direction of a "negative identity," with subsequent alienation and acting out in adolescence. Family dialogue about adoption that is neither perfunctory nor excessive should be encouraged, and by means of which the child can find a way to connect inner fantasies with real surroundings.

When adoptees have difficulty in childhood or adolescence it is often in the form of problems with aggression and impulse control. Many are considered hyperactive and given medication. This is sometimes appropriate, but a more psychodynamic approach may be in order.

Extended psychotherapy is often needed, and the parents need access to the child's therapist perhaps more than do nonadoptive parents because of their own vulnerability to feelings of guilt and decreased self-esteem. In other situations, a case-management approach is useful.

Clinicians should be alert to parents who stonewall the topics of adoption and infertility, because children in such families often feel foreclosed from an important part of their personal histories. Often much help is needed in these families.

Tertiary Intervention

Some adolescent adoptees suffer long-standing neurotic or characterologic impairment, in whose genesis the fact of their adoption, or the life circumstances surrounding it, play an important part (1, 2, 7, 11).

Adolescent developmental issues involving separation and individuation are particularly hard for some adoptees and their parents to negotiate, and at times families present in states of profound crisis. The child psychiatrist must help the family decide whether outpatient psychotherapy has been given an adequate try in the past, and should now be vigorously pursued, or whether the adolescent and the family need some distance from each other. When feasible, boarding school or some alternative living situation (such as having the teenager live with relatives for a time) is a sanity-saving measure—particularly when the adolescent provokes the parents continually and a battle has been set up in which there are no winners. Under such circumstances, the boy or girl will often do better if given a chance for self-definition in a new peer group and with adults whose approach is warm but relatively impersonal, rather than with parents whose love and concern he or she is not able to make use of at this stage.

Occasionally the degree of mutual hostility is impossible to break through, or the parents are implacably rejecting toward a son or daughter who appears to the clinician to be a manageable teenager. When this occurs and the expedients mentioned above are not available, the psychiatrist may wind up presiding over the break-up of a family. If extrusion of the adolescent seems inevitable, the clinician does best not to fight the emotional realities, but rather should try to help each member of the group understand how things came to be so difficult in the family, to facilitate grieving, and to remain available to parents, adolescents, and siblings in whatever way seems feasible. Referral to a social service is usually appropriate at this point. When teenagers must go into foster-care or group-care, it is important for the therapist to initiate contact with the child's new caretakers; often the teenager will be greatly reassured by this continued manifestation of interest. It is better if continued clinical contact is possible; often such contact represents the most stable continuity in an adolescent's life over a turbulent time.

Conclusion

Although the emotional development of adoptees within their families (especially adoptees with traumatic histories) is often troubled to some extent, the majority do well in the long run. Child psychiatrists can assume an attitude of watchful hopefulness with adoptees and their families, helping them to face difficult issues while maintaining a justified belief that long-standing ties are likely to survive present crises.

Foster Care

Half a million American children are in foster homes (12). Such care may be required transiently or for longer periods; at parents' request, or involuntarily when parents are unable to care for or control a child. Some are eventually placed in group-care facilities.

Removal may occur at so young an age that the child retains no memories. Older children suffer from separations, even when parents are neglectful or abusive. Both groups are traumatized by impersonal treatment, lack of continuity of foster homes and social workers, and lack of connection with families of origin.

Children hope for a reconstituted family, although aware of parental failings. The role-reversals forced on many such children lead to conflict between ego progression and the role-reversed regressions involved in looking out for an impaired parent.

Foster homes have the task of providing emotional support, structure, and caring commitment, while not becoming so invested that they make subsequent planning (e.g., for placement back with natural parents, or in an adoptive home) difficult. The foster parents' attitude toward the natural parents should be helpful rather than competitive, and they should not downgrade them to the child. Ideally they should receive substantial initial training and ongoing supervision as paraprofessionals.

Most are conscientious and well-motivated people selected by social agencies. At times scarce funding and heavy caseloads, however, compromise the quality of agency work. Some foster homes are neglectful, abusive, or overcrowded. Professionals involved with individual children can help agencies in their monitoring function.

Permanency planning refers to existing social policy that encourages early decisions in child placement. Too often in the past, foster children were left in limbo without clear goals on the part of those in charge. Children deserve a permanent home; increasingly this principle displaces that of parental rights. Guidelines include:

- Children should not remain in homes that cannot meet their needs.
- Foster children deserve timely decisions regarding their parents' potential to care for them again.
- If such potential is judged lacking, other plans should be made and put into effect.

Some children do better in long-term foster placement than in adoptive homes, for various reasons. Under certain conditions, foster parents may become adoptive parents for a child in their care. Services to natural parents, including counseling and visitation with the child, are important; in their absence, not only does the child suffer, but subsequent attempts to terminate parental rights become difficult even when appropriate.

Disturbances of foster children arise from early deprivation, subsequent disruption, or both. Many foster children have transient adjustment reactions when placed, including regression in sphincter-control, withdrawal, aggression, and problems with sleep and appetite. Underlying psychological causes include:

- Grief at separation from parents and guilt toward them.
- Anxiety and confusion about what will happen in their lives and when.
- Anger at authorities for disrupting their lives, at foster parents for exerting authority, and at parents for abuse or neglect.
- Lowered self-esteem and depression due to feeling abandoned by parents (whatever the circumstances of removal).

Interventions include:

- *Routine monitoring*. A child psychiatrist who sees a foster child should consider:
  - Does this placement seem to be working for the child? Is there evidence of good care? Are there signs of neglect, or physical or sexual abuse?
  - Is the child likely to return to the family of origin? Are

there criteria for deciding if and when the child should be returned? Are parents being offered appropriate services and visitation?
- Has the child been evaluated adequately from the pediatric, dental, neurologic, cognitive, and emotional standpoints, as may be indicated (13)?
- Is there a clearly formulated treatment plan, including psychotherapy if indicated and a periodic review of progress?
- In the absence of indicators for reunion, are appropriate steps being taken to try to free the child for adoption or to make alternate arrangements such as specialized or long-term foster care or group care?

- *Evaluations* with respect to the child's overall treatment plan. Assessment may be required of an emotional and cognitive status in relation to possible placements (e.g., back with parents, in a specialized foster home, or in group care).
- *Psychotherapy* for reactive or long-standing problems. Continued placement in a foster home may be threatened and the therapist seen as one who may help save it. Therapy is often an essential lifeline for a foster child. Even at a time of turmoil, when therapy cannot accomplish structural changes in personality, it can serve as an important stabilizing force.

Children in group homes have much in common with foster children. Many have been in both kinds of settings. These children have an importance disproportionate to their numbers because they represent the most deprived and volatile segment of the child population. Group-care facilities often have access to child psychiatric consultation, but only the best of them provide regular psychotherapy for the children in their care.

Conclusion

Children living in substitute care form a continuum. At one end are group homes; at the other, adoption with the formation of permanent bonds. The themes of abandonment, loss, and diminished self-esteem pertain to all such children to some degree.

References

1. Schechter MD, Carlson PV, Simmons JQ, et al: Emotional problems in the adopted. Arch Gen Psychiatry 10:109–118, 1964

2. Brinich P: Some potential effects of adoption on self and object representations. Psychoanal Study Child 35:107–133, 1980

3. Dukette R: Value issues in present-day adoption. Child Welfare 53:223–243, 1984

4. Blum H: Adoptive parents: generative conflict and generational continuity. Psychoanal Study Child 38:141–163, 1983

5. Kirk HD: Shared Fate: A Theory of Adoption and Mental Health. New York, Free Press, 1964

6. Schechter MD: About adoptive parents, in Parenthood: Its Psychology and Psychopathology. Edited by Anthony EJ, Benedek T. Boston, Little, Brown and Co, 1970

7. Sorosky AD, Baran A, Pannor R: The Adoption Triangle. Garden City, New York, Anchor Books, 1979

8. Rutter M: Maternal Deprivation Reassessed (2d ed). New York, Penguin, 1981

9. Goldstein J, Freud A, Solnit, AJ: Beyond the Best Interests of the Child. New York, Free Press, 1979

10. Derdeyn AP, Levy AM, Looney JG, et al: Child Custody Consultation: Report on the Task Force on Clinical Assessment in Child Custody. Washington, DC, American Psychiatric Association, 1982

11. Nickman SL: Losses in adoption. Psychoanal Study of the Child 40:365–398, 1985

12. Geiser RL: The Illusion of Caring: Children in Foster Care. Boston, Beacon Press, 1973

13. Schor EL: The foster care system and health status of foster children. Pediatrics 69:521–528, 1982

Chapter 15

Infant and Toddler Psychiatry

Margaret P. Gean, M.D.

Child psychiatrists have been intrigued with infants and toddlers for most of the twentieth century. Such noted clinicians and researchers as Winnicott, Spitz, Bowlby, Anna Freud, Mahler, and Klein have contributed to present-day enthusiasm and investigation. It is essential for the child psychiatrist to be aware of the volume of data available that delineates the unique and complex capacities of this age group. It is no longer sufficient to evaluate a very young child solely by speaking with the parent and observing the child. Signs and symptoms of autism, mental retardation, gender disorders, failure-to-thrive, abuse, anxiety disorders, developmental deviations, and reactive disorders may be identified and treated. Children with vulnerabilities to major mental illness may need to be monitored and have early symptomatic treatment. Additionally, difficulties in parenting styles warrant attention as early as possible to prevent dysfunctional parent–child relationships as well as primary psychiatric illness in the child (1–9).

Evaluation

To formulate a diagnosis and treatment plan, several appointments are usually needed, whether the child is seen as an outpatient or while hospitalized (10–11). An initial interview with the parents alone is optimal; talking candidly in the presence of all but the youngest infant may be disturbing to the child. Further, it is difficult for a parent to focus on the evaluator's detailed questions while simultaneously attending to the child's needs. Occasionally parents feel such urgency in having the child seen or are too anxious to talk with the doctor without the child present that this order may have to be modified.

It should also be noted that the presence of the child for some of the interviews will stimulate further information from parents as well as provide for observations of the child and the parent–child relationship. This phase is essential to the evaluation and will be described in detail later.

If a parent must always bring the child or young siblings to the appointment, prior baby-sitting arrangements should be made to ensure that the parent may be talked with in private without leaving the children unsupervised or further stressed by separation from adults with whom they are familiar. The chief complaint; expectations of the evaluation; details of the pregnancy, labor, and delivery; and the medical history of the child should be covered.

Maximum data about the chief complaint is helpful in formulating the diagnosis and treatment as well as in clarifying the style and degree of parental involvement with the child. Such information as when, how long, after what, how frequently, and the details of external circumstances should be inquired about if not provided spontaneously. A description of the personality of the child and the parents' theory as to the etiology of the problem should be elicited. Ages of the accomplishment of developmental landmarks (smiling, sitting, self-feeding, first words, separation anxiety, walking, toilet training), history of parent–child separations, and precipitants of affective responses such as anger and sadness are essential data. One should also gather information concerning the child's daily schedule of meals, naps, sleep patterns, toileting, and play activities (see references 2, 6, 7, 8, and 12 for more information about the expectable ages for these landmarks and descriptions of social, emotional, and attachment development). Inquiries into the parents' own life is warranted; current family stress, recent pregnancy, miscarriage, and history of trauma (e.g., loss of parent, abuse, depressed parent, illness, separation) in the parents' own younger years may elucidate why a parent is having difficulty parenting during a particular developmental phase.

A second appointment should be scheduled at an optimal time for the child (i.e., not nap time or meal time or, in general, late in the day). General observations of the child begin in the waiting room and should include the child's response to any unfamiliar people present and the introduction of the evaluator.

The parents' interactions with the child should be noted, such as the quality with which the child is held, whether eye contact is made, can the parents engage the child in socially reciprocal interchanges, and how do they attend to the child's response to the strange environment. Feeding and diapering may be observed during the evaluation process and permission should be given to the parent to do these tasks as necessary while the evaluator observes.

An assessment of an infant or toddler requires that the evaluator develop a standard format of "interviewing." As language and elaborative fantasy play are limited, a broad array of interactions must be elicited. An opportunity to evaluate the child's social skills, emotional development, degree of primary attachment, cognitive level, language progression, motor skills, physical development, and personality is necessary. The basic circumstances that will allow for systematic assessment of these capacities are the following:

- History from parents or other primary caregiver
- Observation of parent-child interaction in structured and unstructured play
- Observation of child in independent, structured, and unstructured play

- Observation of child's interaction with the evaluator in structured and unstructured tasks
- Developmental assessment (Bayley Scales of Infant Development or Denver Developmental Screening Test)
- Child's response to a brief separation and reunion with the parent
- Review of medical records including birth records

Given the developmental needs of young children for a sense of security in stressful circumstances, the entirety of an infant–toddler evaluation is carried out with a parent (primary attachment figure) present. Data collected without the parent present is by definition incomplete and may distort or make an accurate diagnosis impossible. A decrease of vocalizing is common for young children under mild stress and should not be misinterpreted as mutism or delay. Free play at the end of a session will often facilitate vocalizing if it has not previously been demonstrated. In addition to test items, other toys that cover the full age-range should be readily at hand:

- Small rattle (safe for mouthing)
- Ball (stuffed or soft to prevent injury or breakage with throwing)
- Pull toy
- Blocks (8–10 will suffice)
- Toy telephone or other item with motion and noise
- Doll or stuffed animal

Such toys will help the parent and child feel comfortable as well as facilitate unstructured play observations. In general, asking the parent to help the child be comfortable in the unfamiliar setting will initiate a parent–child interaction. At this point, if not already occurring, the parents can be asked to allow the child to play independently.

Depending on the age, temperament, and presenting problems of the child, the child psychiatrist can alternately move to a structured interaction with the child—using a developmental scale to assess cognitive, language, motor, and behavior skills—or progress more casually with less structured play activity using nontest toys. The latter option is often necessary with children during phases of stranger anxiety or when there is hesitancy toward the evaluator. Such hesitancy may be reflective of anxiety or distrust on the part of the parent and can usually be alleviated by having the child observe (hear) a comfortable verbal interchange between the parent and the doctor. Positioning the child in the parent's lap or visual field is usually helpful in reducing discomfort. If a child cannot be comforted adequately for evaluation, the interview should be terminated and rescheduled. The evaluator should inquire about the best time for the rescheduled appointment, who should come, and why the parent thinks the child is inconsolable. When sufficient data are not available or when the child cannot be comfortably evaluated, the evaluator should wonder whether the child's primary caregiver (attachment object) may be another person than the one who accompanied the child for the evaluation. This is particularly frequent when dealing with adolescent parents, foster parents, and custodial matters. A grandmother, adult child of a foster parent, father, or live-in babysitter may be the primary attachment figure but not the legally designated parent. Having all caretakers come for the evaluation will usually clarify this point and allow for completion of the evaluation.

The choice of a standardized test to measure cognitive and motor development should vary depending on the needs and interests of the child psychiatrist. If a screening assessment is needed or if the evaluator infrequently evaluates young children, the Denver Developmental Screening Test is suitable and the most widely used tool (8). If in-depth diagnostic and treatment planning is called for and if the child psychiatrist anticipates seeing many young children, the Bayley Scales of Infant Development would be preferable and are widely used for both clinical and research purposes (2). The Bayley scales have been standardized across various economic, ethnic, rural–urban, and sex groupings in the United States and have subsequently been used internationally. Experience through testing a number of children of various ages is essential in developing one's skill and familiarity with this tool. If neither standard tool is available, a repetitive structured approach to interacting with young children during part of the interview will allow the clinician to develop his or her own internally comparative scale. Winnicott (13) outlined the rationale for this approach.

After completion of the structured and unstructured observations and interactions, a direct observation of a separation and reunion of the child and the primary caregiver is warranted. As reported by Ainsworth (12) in a detailed description of the procedure and research, the response of the child on separation and more clearly on reunion provides significant data about the security of the child's attachment to the parent. From a practical standpoint, placing the separation and reunion at the end of the appointment prevents interference with other aspects of the evaluation; the stress from the separation is often significant.

To initiate this task, the parent is asked to leave the office for a brief period and to wait outside the closed door. If more than one caregiver is present, a separation–reunion event should be carried out with each adult–child combination. Have all but the designated adult wait in the reception area until it is his or her turn. This will allow the child psychiatrist to compare the child's differential reaction to each adult separately. The child psychiatrist should observe both the parents' method of departure from the child and the child's response. Children with both age-appropriate and heightened (age-inappropriate) separation anxiety may show immediate distress. Other securely attached children may have a delayed reaction or only look to the door or point or approach the place where the parent had been sitting. Older and unattached children may appear not to have noticed the parents' departure and continue to play (this is also observed if the person leaving the room is not the primary attachment figure). Several minutes should elapse prior to reunion to observe the child's response of delayed distress or self-soothing techniques after immediate distress. The child psychiatrist should be certain the child's immediate response to reunion can be observed and should note three major distinguishing patterns:

- The child who shows no reaction to the return of the parent;

- The child who makes brief contact in some form (e.g., tactile, visual, vocal) and returns to play or test items; and
- The child who actively avoids or is intensely angry at the parent or has sustained contact and no re-engagement in play.

The first of these patterns is likely to reflect a child with a lack of attachment to the person who left the room. The second group of responses can be expected from children with secure attachments to the parent. The third group is associated with ambivalently and insecurely attached children. It should be noted that some children will demonstrate attachment behavior toward strangers or the evaluator (e.g., approaching, physical contact, and clinging). This must be distinguished from the quality of the emotional attachment to a parent described in a separation–reunion event. This attachment behavior is not reflective of a primary emotional attachment to the stranger and is frequently seen in children who have either ambivalent or absent reunion responses during the evaluation.

Before the evaluation is completed, the child's birth records and pediatric evaluation (including growth chart), as well as any prior medical, psychiatric, and social service records, must be reviewed. Essential information may be inadvertently overlooked or not known to a parent during the history taking. Additionally, distortion of information obtained by parents during stress (e.g., labor and delivery, emergency room visits, or prior psychiatric evaluations) and reported during the evaluation may be misleading for the physician. Permission to obtain these records should be requested in writing at the first appointment and ideally reviewed prior to seeing the child. Thus any further details or additional information may be gathered from the parents. (In custodial or foster care circumstances, take care to have the release of information signed by the authorized legal custodian. This is often other than the primary caregiver).

In screening assessments or when it is known that the child will be referred elsewhere for treatment (often closer to home), the child psychiatrist with extensive clinical experience and optimal evaluation circumstances may be able to formulate the problem and discuss interventions with the parent at the end of the second appointment. As previously, arrangements should be made to speak with the parents about the assessment without the child present. A third appointment is optimal, however, and can include further brief observations of the child, the inclusion of observations of both parents or other people (siblings) with the child, and further testing if it is incomplete due to previous sleepiness or hunger of the child or anxiety of a parent.

In describing one's conclusions of an evaluation, it is important to describe the unique strengths and weaknesses of the child accurately. Covering the areas of social, emotional, motor, physical, cognitive, language, and attachment will give parents and other clinicians a comprehensive picture. A difficulty in assessing young children is the complexity and rapidly changing nature of their manifestations of "normal" development. Hence what may be appropriate behavior at one age may not be appropriate at a later time. Describing these findings in terms of "delay" as well as the approximate developmental age of the child (i.e., chronologic age of 12 months, mental development of 9 months of age) is more useful clinically and helps parents to adjust their expectations of the child more effectively than the use of diagnostic labels and test scores (e.g., "mental retardation" and "Mental Development Index-71"). Additionally, the child psychiatrist must note whether the development is progressing in a "normal" pattern but at a slower or faster rate than the chronological age would indicate or whether the pattern is "deviant" and not appropriate at any age (e.g., social impairments of a depressed or autistic child, motor tics, language processing problems, or articulation problems). Given that the test scores of motor and mental development are not predictive of future levels of the child's functioning, the child psychiatrist would be most accurate to talk about a particular area of development as:

- being ahead or delayed by a specific number of months, progressing in the range expected for the child's chronologic age,

- being deviant but not delayed, or
- being deviant in one area, delayed in another, and age-appropriate in others

rather than talking about a child being "bright," "slow," or "normal."

It should be noted that when reporting the results of evaluations for children born prematurely, correction for gestational age may be needed. In general, an infant who has been up to 4 weeks premature without medical complications may need correction of developmental landmarks up until about a year of age. Infants with greater than 4 weeks prematurity not only may have a greater incidence of neurologic damage but may take years to approximate chronologically age-appropriate development. A further note in assessing premature infants is the more passive, less sociable temperament of early infancy. Hence parents may need to be counseled to adjust their expectations of the behavior of the premature infant (14).

DIAGNOSIS

Throughout the evaluation the child psychiatrist is constantly developing hypotheses and attempting to understand the meaning and origin of the presenting problem. The complexity of most situations warrants uninterrupted time (without the patient waiting) for the physician to review and integrate all of the data, score the test materials, and formulate a diagnosis and treatment plan. At the present time, there is no satisfactory, widely accepted nosology for use in diagnosing infants and toddlers. *The Diagnostic and Statistical Manual of Mental Disorders, Third Edition (DSM-III)* (15) has a section of childhood categories, but these are generally inadequate to describe, treat, and make prognostic predictions for very young children. (Useful descriptions of particular symptoms and approaches to formulating diagnoses can be found in references 1, 4, and 7.)

There is little correspondence between symptom choice and etiology in infants and toddlers. For example, a child with an attachment disorder in the relationship with the primary caretaker may present with symptoms suggestive of organic illness or developmental delays. Children with prematurity may appear to have common symptoms of attachment disorders, such as gaze aversion and passivity. Likewise, such common presenting complaints as sleep disturbances, eating disturbances, temper tantrums, and toileting problems have an extensive differential diagnosis from organic origins to emotional conflict. Even when the problem is deemed to have external stressors and occurs in a child who is constitutionally and physically capable of healthy development, there is still a lack of one-to-one correspondence between etiology and symptom formation.

Careful observations in all areas of development and an ability to consider combinations of constitutional, interactional, intrapsychic, environmental, and physiologic contributants to a problem make it feasible to describe the nature of the difficulties and to develop a treatment plan. *DSM-III* Axis I has some categories available that do apply to very young children (e.g., anxiety, attachment, oppositional, eating, posttraumatic, and pervasive developmental disorders). A list of the presenting symptoms may be used to describe further the nature of an infant and toddler's problem. Additionally, on Axis II, there is a specific developmental disorder of language. Mental retardation is an Axis I diagnosis and may be used to describe children progressing in a delayed fashion in many developmental areas. A notation can be used to describe whether this diagnosis is suspected to be on an organic basis (e.g., fetal alcohol syndrome, chromosomal abnormality, perinatal compromise) versus environmental difficulties and a lack of stimulation. Not uncommonly, young children will need multiple diagnostic impressions to describe their problems. For example, a child with a history of medical problems, hospitalizations, prematurity, and congenital anomalies could also have an attachment disorder and mental retardation. Growth failure and malnutrition could be the presenting symptom, with a question being raised as to an organic or a psychosocial cause for the growth failure (e.g., attachment disorder). On the other hand, posttraumatic syndromes may be diagnosed in children with trauma such as facial dog bites, physical or sexual abuse, and other extraordinary events that have exceeded the child's age-limited capacity to master intense emotional stress. In cases of suspected physical and sexual abuse, a physical examination is essential to rule out fractures, infections, and soft-tissue injury. A negative physical examination does not, however, rule out the occurrence of abuse. The use of dolls and pictures to convey information, posttraumatic play, and details repeated to several people can support one's clinical suspicion of abuse and aid in diagnosis and intervention to ensure the child's safety.

Although there is little information presently available, affective disorders should be considered in young children whose presentations approximate the *DSM-III* descriptive criteria (adjusted for age), especially in the presence of a family history of major mental illness. Because a combination of genetic and environmental factors may contribute to symptom formation in schizophrenia, the findings of developmental deviations in infants of schizophrenic parents make it appropriate to provide early clinical interventions. These deviations, however, are not always predictive of schizophrenia but may include other childhood disturbances; consultation with the parents regarding risk factors should take this into account.

Infants and toddlers may have adjustment disorders in response to external stresses. These can occur as the result of life stresses that exceed the age-adjusted emotional and cognitive capacities of young children. Additionally, the lack of an empathetic response of a parent to a usual stress such as the arrival of a sibling, a move, parental stress, or physical illness may result in symptoms. The *DSM-III* "V" codes include a number of categories that are useful in describing family circumstances and the use of *DSM-III* Axis 4 and Axis 5 provides the clinician with a system for categorizing the degree of severity of a child's difficulties and functioning.

TREATMENT

Intervention for the vast array of symptoms in infants and toddler must be based on the etiology of the signs and symptoms as well as on the intensity of the symptoms:

- Direct intervention to child
  - Individual psychotherapy
  - Individual cognitive or sensorimotor stimulation
  - Group intervention
  - Hospitalization
  - Placement

- Indirect intervention via parent
  - Parent guidance and education
  - Psychotherapy of parent—verbal, pharmacologic, hospitalization
  - Case management and concrete services

- Dyadic parent–child intervention
  - Multiple times per week center-based program (often includes education of mother, group activities of parents, parents and children, children with peers, social services, medical care)
  - Once or twice weekly counseling and role modeling in home or in clinic (often using video feedback and developmental assessments to assist parent with information)
  - Day care with parent present some of the time

Treatment ranges from individual counseling of the parents to assist them in dealing with the difficulties to direct individual work with the infant or toddler. Varying combinations of both of these approaches are usually undertaken with young children as well as using group treatment with parent groups and parent–child groups. Both regular and therapeutic day care centers that include involvement with the parents may be able to incorporate particular suggestions from the consulting child psychiatrist. Specific problem-focused therapies can be designed for children with cognitive delays, visual and hearing impairments, or medical problems requiring special treatments. These usually utilize an extensive multidisciplinary and multiagency intervention. Additionally, changes in the child's environmental circumstances and protection from physical abuse and neglect are part of recommendations available to a child psychiatrist. Children who are particularly at risk for disturbances because of emotional, medical, and environmental compromises may require on-going, supportive services to provide constant adjustments to the treatment plan to maximize their opportunity for optimal healthy development. Programs that offer outreach and case management to assist parents in utilizing other services such as pediatric care, day care, and social services may be warranted in addition to psychotherapy. Psychopharmacology for young children is infrequent but may be an adjunct while other interventions take hold (e.g., antihistamines for sedation). Most other common medications for older children and adults are not approved in the first 3 years of life and criteria for their efficacy are presently unknown.

In conclusion, evaluation, diagnosis, and treatment of children from birth to 3 years of age provide an opportunity to assist the family in a direct and preventive way more often than at later stages of development. The child psychiatrist has a chance to draw on the breadth of his or her medical training and the challenge of a unique piece of detective work with each child and family. Interventions call on dynamic, psychotherapeutic, and family therapy skills in addition to leadership and consultation liaison. It is hoped that child psychiatrists will be encouraged to learn the details of normal development of very young children so as to maximize the use of their skills.

REFERENCES

1. Anthony EJ, Koupernik C: The Child in His Family, Vol. 3. New York, John Wiley & Sons, 1973

2. Bayley N: Bayley Scales of Infant Development. New York, The Psychological Corp, 1969

3. Call JD: Helping infants cope with change. Early Child Development and Care 3:229–247, 1974

4. Call JD, Galenson E, Tyson R (eds): Frontiers of Infant Psychiatry, Vol. 1. New York, Basic Books, 1985

5. Call JD, Galenson E, Tyson R (eds): Frontiers of Infant Psychiatry, Vol. 2. New York, Basic Books, 1985

6. Greenspan S: Psychopathology and Adaptation in Infancy and Early Childhood. New York, International Universities Press, 1981

7. Noshpitz JD (ed.): Basic Handbook of Child Psychiatry. New York, Basic Books, 1979

8. Osofsky JD (ed.): The Handbook of Infant Development. New York, John Wiley and Sons, 1979

9. Sherman M: The neonatal intensive care unit. Psychiatr Clin North Am 5:433–443, 1982

10. Gaensbauer TJ, Harmon RJ: Clinical Assessment in Infancy Utilizing Structured Playroom Situations. J Am Acad Child Psychiatry 20:264–280, 1981

11. Minde K, Minde R: Infant Psychiatry. Developmental Clinical Psychology and Psychiatry Series, Vol. 4. Beverly Hills, Calif, Sage Publications, 1986

12. Ainsworth MD: Patterns of Attachment: A Psychological Study of the Strange Situation. Hillsdale, NJ, Lawrence Erlbaum Associates, 1978

13. Winnicott DW: The Observation of Infants in a Set Situation, Through Paediatrics to Psycho-Analysis. New York, Basic Books, 1975

14. Brazelton B, Als H: A new model of assessing behavioral organization in pre-term and full-term infants. J Am Acad Child Psychiatry 20:239–263, 1981

15. American Psychiatric Association: Diagnostic and Statistical Manual of Mental Disorders, 3rd ed. Washington, DC, American Psychiatric Association, 1980

Chapter 16

Genetic Issues in Child Psychiatry

Bonnie D. Cummins, M.Ed.

Kenneth S. Robson, M.D.

Until recently the child psychiatrist's core knowledge of clinical genetics was generally limited to some appreciation of the inheritance of major mental illness. Currently, however, the increasingly numerous and sophisticated studies in this area make familiarity with genetic influences in certain conditions more essential. The purpose of this chapter is to summarize existing areas of genetic knowledge and concerns so that the child psychiatrist can respond as consultant to concerned parents, adolescents, and young adults who may wish to marry, and to clinicians in other specialties (e.g., pediatrics, general psychiatry).

Almost every illness and syndrome in child psychiatry has been subjected to genetic scrutiny. Those most frequently encountered from this perspective include:

- Prediction of adult-onset major mental illness (e.g., schizophrenia, affective disorders)
- Prediction of childhood-onset major mental illness (e.g., autism, Tourette's syndrome, schizophrenia, major depression)

- Prediction of certain syndromes of mental retardation (e.g., Downs syndrome, Prader-Willi syndrome)

In relation to the above, the child psychiatrist as genetic counselor or consultant must be *extremely cautious* in conveying information to parents, their families, propective parents, and consultees. Even in adult onset schizophrenia, the most extensively studied illness from a genetic point of view, controversy over gene–environment interactions and influences continue. In the search for certainty, particularly within the medical model, premature assignment of primary genetic causes for most conditions should be avoided.

GENETIC MECHANISMS

Three categories of genetic defects have been identified in humans: the single mutant gene, multifactorial inheritance, and chromosomal abnormalities.

Patterns of single mutant gene inheritance include a person *heterozygous* for that gene (the mutant exists on only one chromosome of a pair) or *homozygous* for the gene (the mutant exists on both chromosomes of a pair). If the mutant gene has an effect in the heterozygous state it is *dominant*; in the homozygous state it is *recessive*. The four varieties of mutant gene inheritance include:

- Autosomal Recessive: The child of two heterozygous parents has a 25 percent chance of being homozygous; males and females are affected with equal frequency and all offspring of the affected are heterozygous ("carriers"). Common examples are adrenogenital syndrome, Hurler syndrome, phenylketonuria, and Tay-Sachs disease.
- Autosomal Dominant: Both males and females are affected; transmission occurs from one parent to a child and the risk of inheritance is 50 percent for each child. Common examples include achondroplastic dwarfism and Huntington's chorea.
- X-linked Recessive: Only males are affected through carrier

females; each daughter of a carrier has a 50 percent chance of being a carrier and each son a 50 percent chance of inheriting the disease. In each pregnancy, the female carrier has a 25 percent chance of having an affected son. Common examples are some hemophilias, retinitis pigmentosa, possible affective disorders (1), and Lesch-Nyhan syndrome.
- X-linked Dominant: Both males and females are affected from generation to generation; all daughters of an affected father will be affected but none of his sons. These conditions are rare and include vitamin D resistant rickets or the syndrome of multiple malformations and possibly affective disorders (1).

Multifactorial inheritance is the result of the additive effect of one or more abnormal genes and environmental factors. The number of genes involved is not known, and few of the environmental factors have been identified. Most features of this inheritance pattern, however, are different from single mutant gene conditions (2). Schizophrenia and probably most other psychiatric conditions appear to follow the multifactorial pattern.

Chromosomal abnormalities have become an increasingly rich area of study as techniques for the culture and visualization of these structures have become more refined. In child psychiatry the most common manifestations of chromosomal abnormalities are some forms of mental retardation (e.g., Downs syndrome, Turner syndrome, and Klinefelter syndrome). Atypical sex chromosome conditions also occur and have been implicated in some behavioral syndromes in childhood; these include the XXX female, the XYY male (implicated in aggressive behaviors), and XX in phenotypic males. The more familiar examples of the mechanics of chromosomal abnormalities are *extra chromosomes* (trisomy 21 or Downs syndrome), *deletions* (cri du chat syndrome), *breakage* ("fragile X syndrome," which may account for up to 30 percent of X-linked mental retardation in males and 10 percent of all mild mental retardation in females), and *translocations* (5 percent of Downs syndrome and unrelated to maternal age).

Risk and Probability in Common Psychiatric Conditions

In the risk statistics presented below, the reader should keep in mind the wide variations in reported percentages and the substantial disagreement among thoughtful students of genetic psychiatry regarding both whether genetic factors play a role in most of these conditions and, if so, precisely how much. For this reason the child psychiatrist as genetic consultant may wish to convey the idea of *probable* or *possible* inherited predispositions of, in most cases, uncertain quantification.

Adult Onset of Major Mental Illness

Schizophrenia (3)

The genetic risk for schizophrenia is outlined in Table 1. In general, most authors favor a polygenic or multifactorial explanation of the genetic influences in schizophrenia.

Affective Disorders (4, 5)

Affective disorders are receiving increasing attention from the genetic perspective. The data are convincing and confusing as well. Certainly, familial–genetic factors seem to be operating across the spectrum of affective conditions. Risk prediction appears to vary with bipolar and unipolar populations and, in some studies, in relation to gender. In the

Table 1. Genetic Risk for Schizophrenia

Affected Relative	Risk to Child (%)
One parent (mother or father)	8–18
Both parents	35–45
Sibling	9–10
Monozygotic twin	40–50
Dizygotic twin	9–10
Second degree relative	2–3

families of anorectic patients, there is a high incidence of both unipolar and bipolar illness, suggesting connections between both disorders.

Direct observation of the offspring of affectively ill parents are gaining momentum (6). Weissman et al. (7), for example, showed that the children of depressives are at increased risk for psychiatric illness in general and major depression in particular at rates three times that of normal probands. This risk increased linearly with both parents ill in contrast to one parent or neither. Current probabilities for affective disorders are shown in Table 2. As in schizophrenia, the most viable model of genetic transmission is multifactorial (polygenic). There are consistent data suggesting a rising influence of genetic factors across the unipolar–bipolar schizoaffective spectrum.

Huntington's Chorea

Although not a major mental illness, per se, this neurological disease is accompanied by serious mental illness, both depression and dementia. It is inherited through a single autosomal dominant gene (50 percent of all offspring of an afflicted parent will contract the disease) but does not become clinically evident until adult life (35–45 years), *after* decisions to marry and bear children have generally been made (8).

Table 2. Genetic Risk for Affective Disorder

Affected Relative	Risk to Child (%)
One parent	27
Both parents	50–74
Monozygotic twin	67*
Dizygotic twin	15*
Second degree relative	2–3

*Bipolar twins appear to have a higher concordance rate than unipolar twins; dizygotic rates are equal for both populations.

Childhood Onset of Major Mental Illness

The data are scantier and less reliable in these conditions. Nevertheless, increasing evidence points to genetic influence in several disorders that include the following:

Infantile Autism (9)

All published reports agree that approximately 2 percent of siblings of autistics are afflicted with infantile autism, a rate 50 times greater than the general population. Further, concordance in monozygotic twins is significantly greater than in dizygotic twins. Nonautistic family members share various language or other cognitive problems with the proband, although of much less severity.

Schizophrenia (10, 11)

This population of children has been surrounded by diagnostic controversy from the outset. There is agreement that children so diagnosed have a higher incidence of schizophrenia in their families than autistics or normal controls. Those twin studies that exist confirm high concordance in monozygotic twins and low concordance in dizygotic twins. Studying infants born to schizophrenic mothers, Fish and Petro (11) believe that the inherited neuro-integrative deficit in schizophrenia is pan-developmental retardation. Finally, many studies support the development of adult schizophrenia in significant numbers of patients diagnosed with both schizophrenia and autism in childhood.

Tourette's Syndrome (12)

It is well documented that this condition evidences both familial concentration and genetic influences. There is significantly higher incidence of tics in the families of afflicted children, suggesting a continuum of genetic vulnerability. Mechanisms for such transmission are unknown.

MAJOR DEPRESSION

Although evidence is accumulating that supports genetic influence in other child psychiatric conditions, including separation disorders, attention deficient disorder, and delinquency, these data have limited clinical usefulness at present. (See "Affective Disorders" above and references 6 and 7).

Mental Retardation (13)

Between 2.3 and 3 percent of the population are defined as mentally retarded (i.e., IQ < 70). Approximately 75 percent of the mentally retarded fall into the "mild" range (50–70 IQ) and this group tends to have no identifiable pathology, higher morbidity, or mortality rates. Genetic influences tend to be nonspecific and probably polygenic (multifactorial). In the population of retarded with IQs less than 50, one-half have disorders of unknown etiology, one-quarter have traumatic/infectious causes, and one-quarter have genetic causes. Within this latter subgroup, 75 percent result from chromosomal abnormalities, 20 percent from single gene disorders, and 5 percent from central nervous system malformations. The conditions most likely to come to the attention of child psychiatrists are listed in Table 3.

Table 3. Inherited Syndromes Associated with Mental Retardation

Syndrome	Mode of Inheritance
Downs syndrome	
94%	Trisomy 21
2.4%	Mosaic
3.6%	Translocation
Tay-Sachs disease	Autosomal recessive
Hurler syndrome	Autosomal recessive
Hunter disease	X-linked recessive
Phenylketonuria	Autosomal recessive
Lesch-Nyhan syndrome	X-linked recessive
Laurence-Moon-Biedl syndrome	Autosomal recessive
Prader-Willi syndrome	Unknown
Fragile X syndrome	X-chromosomal vulnerability

The child psychiatrist's knowledge of these and related conditions is important in:

- differential diagnosis (e.g., infantile autism, hypogenitalism),
- therapeutic interventions with children and their families, and
- genetic counseling of parents or prospective parents (e.g., the differential inheritance of the three types of Downs syndrome).

Conclusion

The technologies for the study, diagnosis, and treatment of genetically caused or influenced illness are increasingly complex. Careful family study, amniocentesis, tissue culture techniques, and basic research into gene (RNA/DNA) structure represent separate disciplines in their own right (2). Furthermore, the identification of "genetic markers" that allow prenatal or childhood diagnosis of adult onset diseases (possibly depression and Huntington's chorea [8]) raises new and complicated questions of both medico–legal and ethical kinds. The child psychiatrist faced with such questions must become well informed through consultation with other professionals. If, for example, 5 percent of the population is at genetic risk for schizophrenia (probably a multifactorial illness) but only 1 percent become clinically ill, what effect would prenatal identification of a genetic marker have in shifting a child (in adult life) into health? Problems of this complexity will confront child psychiatrists in the future with increasing frequency. Closer collaboration with medical colleagues will accelerate mastery of the genetic knowledge base and its accompanying clinical skills.

References

1. Gershon ES: Nonreplication of linkage to X chromosome markers in bipolar illness. Arch Gen Psychiat 37:1200, 1980

2. Nelson WE, Behrman RE, Vaughan VC (eds): Textbook of Pediatrics, 12th ed. Philadelphia, WB Saunders Co, 1983

3. Weiner H: Schizophrenia: etiology, in Comprehensive Textbook of Psychiatry IV, Vol 1. Edited by Kaplan HI, Sadock BJ. Baltimore, Williams & Wilkins, 1985, pp 650–680

4. Rainer JD: Genetics and psychiatry, in Comprehensive Textbook of Psychiatry IV, Vol 1. Edited by Kaplan HI, Sadock BJ. Baltimore, Williams & Wilkins, 1985, pp 25–42

5. Gershon ES, Nurnberger JI, Berrettini WH, et al: Affective disorders: genetics, in Comprehensive Textbook of Psychiatry IV, Vol 2. Edited by Kaplan HI, Sadock BJ. Baltimore, Williams & Wilkins, 1985, pp 778–786

6. Beardslee WR, Bemporad J, Keller MB, et al: Children of parents with major affective disorder. Am J Psychiatry 140:825–832, 1983

7. Weissman MM, Prussoff BA, Gammon GD, et al: Psychopathology in the children of depressed and normal parents. J Am Acad Child Psychiatry 23:78–84, 1984

8. Bird SJ: Presymptomatic testing for Huntington's disease. JAMA 253:3286–3291, 1985

9. Campbell M, Green WH: Pervasive developmental disorders of childhood, in Comprehensive Textbook of Psychiatry IV, Vol 2. Edited by Kaplan HI, Sadock BJ. Baltimore, Williams & Wilkins, 1985, pp 1672–1683

10. Stabeneau JR: Some genetic and family studies in autism and childhood schizophrenia, in Mental Health in Children, Vol 1. Edited by Sankar DVS. Westbury, NY, PJD Publications Ltd, 1975, pp 31–60

11. Fish B, Petro ER: Psychoses of childhood, in Basic Handbook of Psychiatry, Vol 2. Edited by Noshpitz J. New York, Basic Books, 1979, pp 249–304

12. Pauls DL, Kruger SD; Leckman JE, et al: The risk of Tourette's syndrome and chronic multiple tics among relatives of Tour-

ette's syndrome patients obtained by direct interview. J Am Acad Child Psychiatry 23:134–137, 1984

13. Szymanski LS, Crocker AC: Mental retardation, in Comprehensive Textbook of Psychiatry IV, Vol 2. Edited by Kaplan HI, Sadock BJ. Baltimore, Williams & Wilkins, 1985, pp 1635–1671

Index

Academic skills, 73–74
  assessment, 78–81
  curricular progression, 74–78
Acute dystonic reaction, 175
Adoption
  consultation, 247
  overview, 269–270
  personality development factors, 270–271
  post-placement assessment, 278–283
  process related interventions, 271–277
Affective disorders, 306
Affect/mood, 31
Age equivalency (AE) score, 73
Agency consultation, 247–248
Agency referrals, 25–26
Aggression, 192–195
Alcoholic sexual offenders, 233–234
Alprazolam, 169
Ambulatory EEG recording, 44–45
Ammons Quick Test, 71
Anorexia, 207
Anticonvulsants, 174
Antidepressants, 155, 163, 166
Antihistamines, 166, 169

Antiparkinsonian agents, 174–175
Antipsychotic drugs, 155, 158, 161, 175
Anxiolytics, 166, 169–170, 202, 205–206
Appearance and behavior, 31
Apperception tests, 90–91
Attention deficit disorders (ADD), 5, 105–106, 161–162
Audiological screening, 36, 37
Autism, 308

Barbiturates, 206
Bayley Scales of Infant Development, 293
Behavior therapy, 131, 141–143
Bender-Gestalt test, 83–84
Benzodiazepines, 169, 206
β-adrenergic blockers, 175, 178
Blacky Pictures test, 91
Blood chemistry studies, 42
Brain electrical activity monitoring (BEAM), 45
Bulimic anorexia nervosa, 207

Case history, 10–14
Case monitoring, 264–266, 285–286
CAT scanning, 42–43
Child abuse, 197–200
Child interviews, 30–33, 222, 224–230
Children's Apperception Test (CAT), 90–91
Children's drawings, 84–86, 89
Children's rights, 252–254
Chloral hydrate, 169
Chlordiazepoxide, 169
Chlorpromazine, 205, 206
Chromosomal disorders, 37, 305
Chromosomal studies, 46
Clonidine, 178
Cognitive assessment, 69–73, 99–101, 293
Columbia Mental Maturity Scale, 72
Commitment, 254, 255
Complete blood count (CBC), 41, 155, 157
Computerized axial tomography (CAT), 42–43
Conscience/impulse control, 32
Consent, 156, 252–254
Consultation
  adoption and foster care, 247
  agency, 247–248
  forensic, 247, 261–262
  overview, 243–244
  political, 248–249

Consultation (*continued*)
  process, 244–245
  school, 246–247
Coordination and movement, 31–32
Countertransference, 122–123, 274
Custody placement, 255–256, 258

Day hospitals, 135
Delinquency, 254–255
Denver Development Screening Test, 293
Detroit Test of Learning Aptitude (DTLA), 83, 84
Developmental history, 14–17
Developmental Test of Visual-Motor Integration (VMI), 71
Development process, 3–5
Dexamethasone suppression test, 45–46
Dextroamphetamine, 162
Diagnosis. *See* Differential diagnosis; Formulation
Diagnostic and Statistical Manual of Mental Disorders, Third Edition (DSM-III), 104–106, 298, 299
Diagnostic assessment
  adoption related, 272–277
  case history, 10–14
  child interviews, 30–33, 222, 224–230
  clinical approach, 22–23
  communicating diagnosis and treatment plan, 107–109
  developmental history, 14–17
  differential diagnosis, 104–106
  emergencies, 185–186, 188–190, 193–194, 199
  family interviews, 29–30, 189, 224
  forensic, 258–261
  formulation, 103–104, 190, 234–235, 297–299
  goals of, 21–22
  infants and toddlers, 290–297
  medical model and, 8, 10
  parent interviews, 26–28, 222, 230–234
  psychopathology factors, 3–8
  referral factors, 23–26
  setting for, 17–19
  treatment planning, 106–107, 235, 238–239
  See also Medical evaluation; Psychological testing
Diazepam, 169
Differential diagnosis, 104–106
Diphenhydramine, 194
Drawing tests, 84–86, 89
Drug abuse, 202–203, 205–206, 253
Drugs. *See* Pharmacotherapy
Dyskinesias, 152–153, 161

Eating disorders, 206–208
Educational experience, 73–81
Education Apperception Test, 91
Ego-relatedness, 7, 127
Electroencephalogram (EEG), 43–45, 155
Emergencies
    aggression, 192–195
    child abuse, 197–200
    consent to treatment and, 252
    eating disorders, 206–208
    homicide, 195–197
    overview, 185–186
    psychosis, 200–206
    school refusal, 208–210
    suicide, 186–191
    See also Sexual abuse
Empathic failure, 5, 7–8, 113, 114
Empirical/objective personality measures, 92–93
Evaluation. *See* Diagnostic assessment
EXAMINS (Examination for Minor Neurological Signs), 40, 57–63
Extended Merrill-Palmer Scale, 71
Extrapyramidal side effects, 158, 175

Family
    drawings, 86
    interviews, 29–30, 189, 224
    therapeutic work, 124
Fantasy, 127
Fetal alcohol syndrome, 37
Financial issues, 26–27, 69, 88, 107
Fixated sexual offenders, 232
Folic acid deficiency test, 42
Forensic child psychiatry
    children's rights, 252–254
    consultation, 247, 261–262
    custody placement, 255–256
    delinquency, 254–255
    evaluation, 258–261
    monitoring, 264–266
    parental rights termination, 256, 258
    report writing, 262–263
    testimony, 263–264
Formulation, 103–104, 190, 234–235, 297–299
Foster care, 247, 284–287
Fragile X syndrome, 37
Functional psychosis, 200–201
Furnishings, 17–19

Games, 127
Genetic issues
  adult onset risks, 306–307
  childhood onset risks, 308
  defect categories, 304–305
  laboratory studies, 46
  major depression, 309–310
  overview, 303–304
Goodenough-Harris Drawing Test, 71
Group for the Advancement of Psychiatry, 104
Group homes, 136, 286
Group therapy, 127–128, 235

Haloperidol, 205, 206
Halstead-Reitan Neuropsychological Battery, 95–96
Haptic Intelligence Test for Adult Blind, 72
Hiskey-Nebraska Test of Learning Aptitude, 72
Homicide, 195–197
Hospital-based treatment, 134–135, 190–191, 194, 199, 203, 207
House/tree/person test, 85–86
Human figure drawings, 85
Huntington's chorea, 307
Hydroxyzine, 194
Hypnosis, 131, 145–147

Imipramine, 163
Incest, 215–216. *See* also Sexual abuse
Incomplete sentence tests, 89
Individual child psychotherapy, 125–127
Infant and toddler psychiatry
  diagnosis, 297–299
  evaluation, 290–292
  treatment, 299–301
Infantile autism, 308
Informed consent, 156, 252–254
Inkblot test, 89–90
Intelligence testing, 69–72
Intensive milieu therapy, 131
  placement factors, 136–138
  principles of, 138–139
  settings for, 134–136
Interviews
  adoption related, 275–277
  child, 30–33, 222, 224–230
  child abuse related, 199
  diagnostic assessment, 26–33

Interviews (*continued*)
  family, 29–30, 189, 224
  infant and toddler, 290–295
  parent, 26–28, 222, 230–234
  referral agency, 25–26
  sexual abuse, 222, 224–234
  suicide related, 189

Juvenile sexual offenders, 234

Kaufman-Assessment Battery for Children, 71
Kinetic family drawings, 86

Laboratory studies
  biochemical, 41–42, 157
  brain electrical activity monitoring, 45
  drug abuse related, 203
  electroencephalogram, 43–45, 155
  neuroendocrinological, 45–46
  predrug work-up, 155–157
  radiological and neuroimaging, 42–43
Legal testimony, 263–264
Leiter International Performance Scale, 72
Lithium, 156, 170, 174
Liver profile, 42, 155
Luria-Nebraska Neuropsychological Battery (Children's Revision), 96

Major depression, 309
McCarthy Scales of Children's Abilities, 71
Medical evaluation
  laboratory studies, 41–46, 155–156
  minor physical anomalies, 37–38
  neurological examination, 39–41, 49–63, 154
  physical examination, 36–37, 154
  predrug work-up, 154–156
  psychiatric disorders and, 35–36
  rape, 236–237
Medical model, 8, 10
Mental age (MA) score, 72–73
Mental retardation, 309
Merrill-Palmer Scale of Mental Tests, 71
Methylphenidate, 162
Minneosota Multiphasic Personality Inventory, 92–93
Minor physical anomalies (MPAs), 37–38
Monitoring, 157, 264–266, 285–286
Monoamine oxidase (MAO), 166
Motor-Free Visual Perception Test, 83

Multifactorial inheritance, 305, 307
Mutant gene inheritance, 304–305

Neuroendocrinological studies, 45–46
Neuroimaging studies, 42–43
Neuroleptics, 155, 158, 161, 175
Neurological examination
  comprehensive procedure, 49–56
  overview, 39–41
  predrug work-up, 154
  psychosis and, 201
  short procedure, 57–63
  See also Laboratory studies
Neuropsychological testing, 93–97
Night terrors, 169
Nuclear magnetic resonance (NMR), 43

Office playroom, 17–19
Open adoption, 274–275
Organic psychoses, 201–203, 205
Orgiastic relatedness, 7
Overstimulation, 5, 7–8, 113, 114

Parents
  child abuse and, 198–200
  drug therapy and, 150–151, 157
  interviews, 26–28, 222, 230–234
  rights termination, 256, 258
  therapeutic work with, 121–124
Peabody Picture Vocabulary Test-Revised, 71
Pediatric consultation-liaison, 245–246
Pemoline, 162
Perception/cognition, 32
Perceptual motor skills, 81, 83–84
Permanency planning, 274, 284–285
Personality assessment. *See* Empirical/objective personality measures;
    Projective assessment
Personality Inventory for Children, 93
PET scanning, 43
Pharmacotherapy
  aggression, 194
  anticonvulsants, 174
  antidepressants, 155, 163, 166
  antiparkinsonian agents, 174–175
  anxiolytics and sedative-hypnotics, 166, 170, 202, 205–206
  drug interactions, 179
  guidelines, 150–153

Pharmacotherapy (*continued*)
  indications for use, 149–150
  infants and toddlers, 301
  lithium, 156, 170, 174
  maintenance and monitoring, 157
  neuroleptic drugs, 155, 158, 161, 175
  predrug work-up, 153–157
  propranolol, 175–176, 206
  psychosis, 203, 205–206
  psychostimulants, 155, 161–163
  side effects, 152, 158, 161, 162, 166, 169–170, 178–179, 202
Phenothiazines, 206
Physical examination, 36–37, 154, 199, 222–223, 236–237
Physostigmine, 205
Pictorial Test of Intelligence, 72
Playroom setting, 17–19
Political consultation, 248–249
Polysomnography, 46
Positron emission tomography (PET), 43
Predrug work-up, 153–157
Progressive Matrices, 72
Projective assessment, 86–87, 154
  indications for use, 87–88
  limitations of, 88
  test types, 88–93
Prolonged EEG recording, 44
Propranolol, 175–176, 206
Psychological testing
  academic skills, 73–81
  children's drawings, 84–86, 89
  cognitive assessment, 69–73, 99–101, 293
  indications for use, 66–67
  infants and toddlers, 293–294
  limitations of, 68–69
  neuropsychological, 93–97
  overview, 65–66
  projective/personality based, 86–93, 154
  visual perceptual motor skills, 81, 83–84
Psychopathic sexual offenders, 233
Psychopathology, 3–8, 113–114
Psychosis, 200–206
Psychostimulants, 155, 161–163
Psychotherapies
  adoption and foster care related, 282, 286
  change mechanisms, 119–120
  family work, 124

group, 127–128
  indication for use, 120–121
  individual, 125–127
  parent factors, 121–124
Psychotic sexual offenders, 233

Radiological studies, 42–43
Rape, 216, 236–239
Referrals, 23–26, 221
Refusal of treatment, 253–254
Regressed sexual offenders, 232–233
Relatedness, 7, 31
Report writing, 262–263
Residential schools, 135
Retarded sexual offenders, 233
Right to refuse treatment, 253–254
Roberts Apperception Test, 91
Rorschach test, 89–90

Schizophrenia, 306, 308
School consultation, 246–247
School refusal, 208–210
Sedative-hypnotics, 166, 169–170
Seizures, 174
Self-concept, 32
Sexual abuse
  characteristics of, 214–215
  clinical issues, 217–220
  formulation and diagnosis, 234–236
  initial interventions, 221–224
  intervention issues, 220
  interviewing techniques, 224
  legal issues, 216–217
  nonabusing parent factors, 222, 230–232
  offender factors, 222, 232–234
  rape, 216, 236–239
  sources of distress, 220–221
  terminology, 215–216
  victim factors, 222, 224–230
Side effects, 152, 158, 161, 162, 166, 169–170, 178–179, 202
Skin conductance test, 46
Sleep studies, 45, 46
Slosson Intelligence Test, 71
Speech and language, 32
Status offenses, 252

Suicide
    diagnostic assessment, 188–190
    disposition of patient, 190–191
    eating disorders and, 207
    overview, 186–188

Tasks of Emotional Development Test (TED), 91–92
Termination of parental rights, 256, 258
Testimony, 263–264
Thematic Apperception Test (TAT), 90
Therapeutic day schools, 136
Therapist-child patient privilege, 252
Thioridazine, 205
Tourette's syndrome, 178, 308
Toxic screen, 203
Tranquilizers. *See* Sedative-hypnotics
Treatment
    behavior therapy, 131, 141–143
    goals, 116
    hypnosis, 131, 145–147
    infants and toddlers, 299–301
    intensive milieu therapy, 131, 133–139
    modality effectiveness, 117
    planning, 106–107, 235, 238–239
    psychotherapies, 113–128
    therapeutic approach, 113–116
    See also Emergencies; Pharmacotherapy; Sexual abuse
Tricyclic antidepressants, 155, 163, 166

Urinary tract studies, 41, 155–157

Vineland Adaptive Behavior Scales, 93
Vision screening, 36–37
Visual Motor Gestalt Test, 83–84
Visual perceptual motor skills, 81, 83–84, 293
VMI test, 83–84

Wechsler scales, 69–71, 83, 84